Balancing Blood Sugar: Natural Supplements for Diabetes and Neuropathy Relief

By

James Caudle

Published   Dec. 2024

ISBN – 9798303721593

All Rights Reserved

Introduction

Diabetes and neuropathy are conditions that touch the lives of millions globally, often leading to chronic pain, discomfort, and a diminished quality of life. The search for effective management strategies extends beyond conventional medicine, leading many to explore the potential of natural supplements. This book emerges as a guiding light in that quest.

In a world where the incidence of diabetes continues to rise—over 422 million adults globally, according to the World Health Organization—the burden of managing the associated complications, such as neuropathy, grows concurrently. Neuropathy affects approximately 50% of diabetic individuals, manifesting as pain, tingling, and numbness, particularly in the extremities. These symptoms can significantly impair daily activities and overall well-being, highlighting the need for comprehensive management approaches.

Pharmaceutical interventions, while essential, often come with their own set of challenges and side effects. It is within this context that the exploration of natural supplements gains prominence. The promise of nature's bounty—vitamins, minerals, herbs, and other compounds—offers a complementary pathway to traditional treatment plans, aiming to not only alleviate symptoms but also enhance overall health.

This book brings together scientific research, practical insights, and holistic approaches to empower readers in their journey towards better health. It delves into the benefits of supplements like alpha-lipoic acid, chromium, magnesium, and herbal allies such as bitter melon and fenugreek, presenting evidence-based information on how these natural substances can support blood sugar regulation and nerve health.

You will find detailed discussions on the mechanisms by which these supplements exert their effects, dosage recommendations, and potential interactions—ensuring you have the knowledge needed to make informed decisions. Additionally, the book emphasizes the importance of integrating these supplements into a balanced lifestyle, including proper diet and regular physical activity, for optimal results.

This book is more than just a collection of supplement profiles; it is a roadmap to achieving a higher quality of life through natural means. It invites you to embrace a holistic perspective, understanding that true health encompasses the physical, emotional, and environmental aspects of our existence.

As you turn the pages, may you be inspired by the potential of nature to heal and invigorate. May this book serve as a beacon of hope, guiding you towards a path of wellness and vitality.

I encourage you to try some of these supplements and test to see if they will work for you, if they don't, try another one on this list. Try Creating a daily stack of different supplements. Test to see if some of these combinations will alleviate your symptoms. A stack to try might be, Gymnema, berberine, nattokinase, K2, and citrulline. Find a good quality Magnesium to take daily. Vanadium, chromium, and copper and needed to unlock the cell, allowing sugar to enter and replenish the cell. Many other supplements are good for reducing the cell resistance, allowing for insulin to work properly. I the author take daily, Magnesium, Turmeric, Ginger, Carnitine, citrulline, astragalus, lions' mane, nattokinase, black seed oil, berberine, D3, K2, potassium, and some other to help balance my blood sugars.

Where to start?
I should not have to write this, however if you are eating garbage, you will have garbage results. Fix your daily diet and watch what you eat. create an exercise routine and strive for 4 times a week.
Start with the essential nutrients, add vanadium, chromium, copper, Vitamin B8, D3, leucine.
Next add a few supplements, such as berberine, Gymnema, turmeric. And then see how you feel and after a few months get your A1C checked to see your progress.

Disclaimer

This book is for general health information only. This book is not to be used as a substitute for medical advice, diagnosis or treatment of any health condition or problem. People should not rely solely on information provided in this guide book for their own health problems. Any questions regarding your own health should be addressed to your own physician or other healthcare provider.

The author makes no guarantee nor express or implied representations whatsoever regarding the accuracy, completeness, timeliness, comparative or controversial nature, or usefulness of any information contained or referenced in this book. The Author does not assume any risk whatsoever for your use of the information contained herein. Health-related information changes frequently and therefore information contained in this book could become outdated, incomplete, or incorrect.

 You are hereby advised to consult with a physician or other professional health-care provider prior to making any decisions, or undertaking any actions or not undertaking any actions related to any health care problem or issue you might have at any time, now or in the future. You the individual are responsible for what you put in your body.

Diabetes and Blood Sugar

Contents

Understanding type 2 diabetes – P. 1

Understanding type 1 diabetes – P. 3

Trans Fats – P.5

Dietary Fiber – P.7

Weight Training – P.9

Acetyl L Carnitine –P.11

Allulose – P.13

Alpha Lipoic Acid – P.15

Apple Cider Vinegar – P.17

Apple Pectin – P.19

Anamu – P.21

Arjuna – P.23

Arnica – P.25

Astragalus – P.27

Barberry – P.29

Bearberry – P.31

Beech – P.33

Berberine – P.35

Beth Root– P.37

Bilberry – P.39

Bitter Melon – P.41

Bitter Root – P.43

Black Seed Oil – P.45

Blue Flag – P.47

Bromelain – P.49

Cayenne Pepper – P.51

Cats Claw – P.53

Ceylon Cinnamon – P.55

Chinese peony – P.57

Chinese Yam – P.59

Chromium – P.61

Chrysanthemum – P.63

Copper – P.65

Creatine – P.67

Dandelion – P.69

Echinacea – P.71

Fenugreek – P.73

Ginger – P.75

Ginkgo Biloba – P.77

Goji Berries – P.79

Green Tea – P.81

Gymnema-Sylvestre – P.83

Hawthorn – P.85

Hydrangea – P.87

Jujube – P.89

Korean ginseng – P.91

Lemon Balm – P.93

Leucine – P. 95

Licorice Root – P.99

Magnesium – P.101

Milk Thistle – P.103

Nattokinase – P.105

Nitrosigine – P.107

NO3-T – P.109

Plantain – P.111

Poria – P.113

Psyllium Husk – P.116

Raspberry extract – P.118

Rehmannia – P.120

Resveratrol – P.122

Schisandra – P.124

Sumac – P.126

THC Marijuana – P.128

Turmeric – P.130

Vanadium – P.132

Vitamin B8 – P. 134

Vitamin D3 – P.138

White Mulberry – P.140

Wormwood – P.142

Neuropathy

Contents

Neuropathy and its connection to diabetes – P. 145

The Myelin Sheath – P. 147

Acetyl L Carnitine - P. 149

Alpha Lipoic Acid – P. 151

Arnica – P. 153

Bearberry – P. 156

Benfotiamine – P. 158

Bitterroot – P. 160

BPC-157 – P. 162

Chinese Peony – P. 164

Chrysanthemum – P. 167

Co-Q-10 – P. 170

Curcumin – P. 172

Dandelion – P. 174

GABA – P. 177

Gamma Linolenic Acid – P. 179

Ginko Biloba – P. 181

Hawthorn – P. 183

L-Arginine – P. 186

L-Citrulline – P. 188

Lions Mane – P. 190

Magnesium – P. 192

N-Acetyl L-Cysteine – P. 196

Omega 3 Fatty Acid – P. 198

Peppermint – P. 200

Plantain – P. 202

Poria – P. 205

Quercetin – P. 208

Sumac – P. 211

TB-500 – P. 214

THC – P. 216

Vitamin B12 – P. 219

Vitamin B6 – P. 221

White Mulberry – P. 223

Sources – P.226

Type 2 Diabetes: Understanding the Condition.

Type 2 diabetes is a chronic condition that affects the way the body processes blood sugar (glucose). It is the most common form of diabetes, accounting for about 90-95% of all diabetes cases[1]. This book is more focused on helping this type of diabetes, but blood sugar management also works for type 1.

What is Type 2 Diabetes?

Type 2 diabetes occurs when the body becomes resistant to insulin or when the pancreas is unable to produce enough insulin[2]. Insulin is a hormone that regulates the movement of glucose into cells, where it is used for energy. In type 2 diabetes, this process is impaired, leading to elevated levels of glucose in the blood (hyperglycemia).

Effects of Type 2 Diabetes

The effects of type 2 diabetes can be widespread and severe if not managed properly. Some of the key complications include:

- **Cardiovascular Disease**: High blood sugar levels can damage blood vessels and the nerves that control the heart, increasing the risk of heart disease and stroke[3].
- **Kidney Damage**: Diabetes can damage the kidneys' filtering system, leading to kidney disease or even kidney failure[4].
- **Nerve Damage (Neuropathy)**: Excess sugar can injure the walls of the tiny blood vessels that nourish nerves, especially in the legs, leading to pain, tingling, or numbness[5].
- **Eye Damage**: Diabetes increases the risk of serious eye conditions, including cataracts, glaucoma, and diabetic retinopathy, which can lead to blindness[6].
- **Foot Damage**: Nerve damage in the feet or poor blood flow increases the risk of various foot complications[7].

How Insulin Resistance Develops

Insulin resistance is a key feature of type 2 diabetes. It occurs when cells in muscles, fat, and the liver start responding poorly to insulin and cannot easily take up glucose from the blood[8]. Here's how insulin resistance typically develops:

- **Genetic Factors**: Genetics play a significant role in the development of insulin resistance. If you have a family history of type 2 diabetes, you are at a higher risk[9].
- **Obesity**: Excess fat, particularly around the abdomen, is a major cause of insulin resistance. Fat cells release inflammatory substances that can reduce the effectiveness of insulin.
- **Physical Inactivity**: Lack of physical activity contributes to insulin resistance. Regular exercise helps cells respond better to insulin.
- **Diet**: A diet high in refined carbohydrates and sugars can lead to spikes in blood sugar and insulin levels, eventually causing insulin resistance.
- **Hormonal Imbalances**: Certain conditions, such as polycystic ovary syndrome (PCOS), can cause hormonal imbalances that contribute to insulin resistance.

Conclusion

Type 2 diabetes is a complex and multifaceted disease that requires careful management to prevent serious complications. Understanding the condition, its effects on the body, and the mechanisms behind insulin resistance is crucial for effective prevention and treatment. Lifestyle changes, such as maintaining a healthy diet, regular physical activity, and weight management, are essential in managing type 2 diabetes and improving overall health.

Type 1 Diabetes: Understanding the Condition

Type 1 diabetes is a chronic autoimmune condition where the body's immune system mistakenly attacks and destroys the insulin-producing beta cells in the pancreas[1]. This results in little to no insulin production, which is crucial for regulating blood sugar levels.

What is Type 1 Diabetes?

Type 1 diabetes, also known as insulin-dependent diabetes, typically develops in children, teenagers, and young adults, although it can occur at any age[2]. Unlike type 2 diabetes, which is often associated with lifestyle factors, type 1 diabetes is primarily caused by genetic and environmental factors that trigger an autoimmune response[3].

How Type 1 Diabetes Acts in the Body

In a healthy individual, the pancreas produces insulin, a hormone that helps glucose enter the cells to be used for energy. In type 1 diabetes, the immune system attacks the beta cells in the pancreas, leading to a significant reduction or complete cessation of insulin production[4]. Without insulin, glucose cannot enter the cells and remains in the bloodstream, causing high blood sugar levels (hyperglycemia).

The lack of insulin leads to several symptoms and complications:

- **Increased Thirst and Urination**: High blood sugar levels cause the kidneys to work harder to filter and absorb the excess glucose. When the kidneys can't keep up, the excess glucose is excreted into the urine, dragging fluids from the tissues, leading to dehydration and increased thirst[5].
- **Weight Loss**: Despite eating more to relieve hunger, people with type 1 diabetes may lose weight because the body cannot use glucose for energy and starts breaking down muscle and fat for fuel[6].
- **Fatigue**: Without enough insulin, the body cannot efficiently use glucose for energy, leading to feelings of fatigue and weakness[7].
- **Diabetic Ketoacidosis (DKA)**: When the body starts breaking down fat for energy, it produces ketones, which can build up to dangerous

levels in the blood, leading to DKA, a potentially life-threatening condition[8].

Differences Between Type 1 and Type 2 Diabetes

While both type 1 and type 2 diabetes involve issues with insulin and blood sugar regulation, they have distinct differences:

- **Cause**: Type 1 diabetes is an autoimmune condition where the immune system destroys insulin-producing cells[2]. Type 2 diabetes is primarily related to insulin resistance, where the body's cells do not respond properly to insulin, often due to lifestyle factors such as obesity and inactivity[9].
- **Age of Onset**: Type 1 diabetes is usually diagnosed in children and young adults, whereas type 2 diabetes typically develops in adults over the age of 45, although it is increasingly seen in younger populations due to rising obesity rates.
- **Insulin Production**: People with type 1 diabetes produce little to no insulin and require insulin therapy for life[4]. In type 2 diabetes, the body still produces insulin, but it is not used effectively, and insulin production may decrease over time[9].
- **Management**: Type 1 diabetes management focuses on insulin therapy, blood sugar monitoring, and lifestyle adjustments[2]. Type 2 diabetes management includes lifestyle changes, oral medications, and sometimes insulin therapy[9].

Conclusion

Type 1 diabetes is a serious autoimmune condition that requires lifelong management with insulin therapy and careful monitoring of blood sugar levels. Understanding the differences between type 1 and type 2 diabetes is crucial for effective treatment and management. While both conditions share some similarities, their causes, age of onset, and treatment approaches differ significantly. With proper management, individuals with type 1 diabetes can lead healthy and fulfilling lives.

Trans Fats

Trans fats, also known as trans fatty acids, are a type of unsaturated fat that have been chemically altered through a process called hydrogenation. This process makes the fat more solid and extends the shelf life of food products. However, trans fats are notorious for their negative health effects, particularly in relation to blood sugar levels and diabetes.

What Are Trans Fats?

Trans fats are found in many processed foods, including baked goods, snack foods, and fried items. They are created by adding hydrogen to liquid vegetable oils to make them more solid. This process not only improves the texture and shelf life of foods but also makes them more stable for frying[1].

How Trans Fats Affect Blood Sugar and Diabetes

- **Insulin Resistance**: One of the most significant impacts of trans fats is their contribution to insulin resistance. Insulin resistance occurs when cells in the body become less responsive to insulin, a hormone that regulates blood sugar levels. This resistance forces the pancreas to produce more insulin to keep blood sugar levels in check, which can eventually lead to type 2 diabetes[2].
- **Inflammation**: Trans fats promote inflammation in the body, which is a key factor in the development of insulin resistance and type 2 diabetes[3]. Chronic inflammation can damage cells and tissues, impairing their ability to respond to insulin.
- **Weight Gain**: Consumption of trans fats is linked to weight gain, particularly abdominal fat. Excess body fat, especially around the abdomen, is a major risk factor for developing insulin resistance and type 2 diabetes[4].
- **Cholesterol Levels**: Trans fats raise levels of LDL (bad) cholesterol and lower levels of HDL (good) cholesterol. High levels of LDL cholesterol can lead to the buildup of plaques in arteries, increasing the risk of cardiovascular diseases, which are common complications of diabetes[5].

Mechanisms Behind Trans Fats and Diabetes

The exact mechanisms by which trans fats contribute to diabetes are complex and multifaceted:

- **Cell Membrane Composition**: Trans fats can incorporate into cell membranes, altering their structure and function. This can impair insulin signaling pathways, making it harder for cells to respond to insulin.
- **Lipid Metabolism**: Trans fats can disrupt normal lipid metabolism, leading to the accumulation of fat in the liver and other tissues. This can further exacerbate insulin resistance.

Reducing Trans Fat Intake

Given the harmful effects of trans fats, it is crucial to minimize their intake. Here are some tips:

- **Read Food Labels**: Check nutrition labels for trans fats and avoid products that contain partially hydrogenated oils.
- **Choose Healthier Fats**: Opt for healthier fats, such as monounsaturated and polyunsaturated fats found in olive oil, nuts, and avocados.
- **Cook at Home**: Preparing meals at home allows you to control the ingredients and avoid trans fats commonly found in processed and fast foods.

Conclusion

Trans fats have a significant negative impact on blood sugar levels and the development of diabetes. By promoting insulin resistance, inflammation, and weight gain, trans fats increase the risk of type 2 diabetes and its complications. Reducing trans fat intake and choosing healthier fats can help manage blood sugar levels and improve overall health.

The Role of Different Fibers in Managing Diabetes

Dietary fiber is a crucial component of a healthy diet, especially for individuals managing diabetes. Fiber is a type of carbohydrate that the body cannot digest, and it plays a significant role in regulating blood sugar levels, improving insulin sensitivity, and promoting overall metabolic health. There are two main types of dietary fiber: soluble and insoluble, each offering unique benefits for diabetes management.

Types of Fiber

- **Soluble Fiber**: Soluble fiber dissolves in water to form a gel-like substance in the digestive tract. This type of fiber helps slow down the absorption of sugar, which can prevent spikes in blood glucose levels after meals. Soluble fiber is also known to lower cholesterol levels, which is beneficial for cardiovascular health—a common concern for people with diabetes[1].

Sources of Soluble Fiber:

- Oats
- Apples
- Citrus fruits
- Barley
- Legumes (such as beans and lentils)
- Psyllium husk

- **Insoluble Fiber**: Insoluble fiber does not dissolve in water and adds bulk to the stool, aiding in regular bowel movements. While it does not directly affect blood sugar levels, it promotes overall digestive health and can help prevent constipation[2].

Sources of Insoluble Fiber:

- Whole grains (such as whole wheat and brown rice)
- Nuts and seeds
- Vegetables (such as cauliflower, green beans, and potatoes)
- Wheat bran

Benefits of Fiber for Diabetes Management

- **Blood Sugar Control**: Fiber, particularly soluble fiber, helps slow the digestion and absorption of carbohydrates, leading to a more gradual rise in blood sugar levels. This can help prevent the sharp spikes and crashes in blood glucose that are common in diabetes[3].
- **Improving Insulin Sensitivity**: High-fiber diets have been shown to improve insulin sensitivity, which is crucial for managing type 2 diabetes. Improved insulin sensitivity means that the body can use insulin more effectively to lower blood sugar levels[4].
- **Weight Management**: Fiber-rich foods are often more filling and can help promote satiety, reducing overall calorie intake. This can be beneficial for weight management, which is an important aspect of diabetes control[5].
- **Cardiovascular Health**: Soluble fiber helps lower LDL cholesterol levels, reducing the risk of cardiovascular disease—a common complication of diabetes. By improving heart health, fiber contributes to better overall health outcomes for people with diabetes.

Incorporating Fiber into the Diet

- **Start Your Day with Fiber**: Choose high-fiber breakfast options such as oatmeal or whole-grain cereals.
- **Add Legumes**: Incorporate beans, lentils, and chickpeas into soups, salads, and main dishes.
- **Snack on Fruits and Vegetables**: Opt for fresh fruits and vegetables as snacks. Apples, berries, and carrots are excellent choices.
- **Choose Whole Grains**: Replace refined grains with whole grains such as brown rice, quinoa, and whole wheat bread.
- **Include Nuts and Seeds**: Add nuts and seeds to your meals or enjoy them as snacks.

Conclusion

Dietary fiber plays a vital role in managing diabetes by helping to control blood sugar levels, improve insulin sensitivity, and support overall health. Both soluble and insoluble fibers offer unique benefits, making it important to include a variety of fiber-rich foods in your diet. As always, it is essential to consult with a healthcare provider or a registered dietitian to tailor dietary recommendations to your individual health needs.

Weight Training and Its Effects on Blood Sugar and Diabetes

Weight training, also known as resistance training, involves exercises that improve muscle strength and endurance by making muscles work against a weight or force. This form of exercise has gained recognition for its numerous health benefits, particularly in managing blood sugar levels and diabetes. This essay explores the mechanisms through which weight training influences blood sugar control and reviews the clinical evidence supporting its use.

Mechanisms of Action

- **Improving Insulin Sensitivity**: Weight training enhances insulin sensitivity, which is crucial for managing type 2 diabetes. When muscles contract during resistance exercises, they increase glucose uptake from the bloodstream without the need for additional insulin[1]. This improved insulin sensitivity helps lower blood sugar levels and makes the body more efficient at using insulin.
- **Regulating Blood Sugar Levels**: Weight training can help regulate blood sugar levels by increasing muscle mass. More muscle mass means a greater capacity to store glucose as glycogen, which helps stabilize blood sugar levels[2]. Additionally, resistance training can reduce the amount of visceral fat, which is associated with insulin resistance and higher blood sugar levels[3].
- **Reducing Inflammation and Oxidative Stress**: Chronic inflammation and oxidative stress are significant contributors to the development and progression of diabetes. Weight training has been shown to reduce markers of inflammation and oxidative stress[4]. By mitigating these factors, weight training can improve overall metabolic health and prevent complications associated with diabetes.

Clinical Evidence

everal studies have demonstrated the efficacy of weight training in managing diabetes. For instance, a study published in the Journal of Endocrine Society found that participants with type 2 diabetes who engaged in regular weight training showed significant improvements in blood sugar control and insulin sensitivity[5]. Another study highlighted that weight training reduced the risk of developing type 2 diabetes by 32% in individuals at high risk[2].

Moreover, a 2023 study found that participants with type 2 diabetes who did strength training alone showed more improvements in blood sugar levels than those who did cardio alone[4]. This suggests that weight training can be particularly effective for blood sugar management.

Frequency

The American Diabetes Association recommends that adults engage in at least two sessions of strength training per week[3]. It is important to start with a weight that is manageable and gradually increase the intensity to avoid injury. Proper form and technique are crucial to prevent strain and injury. Consulting with a healthcare provider or a certified fitness trainer can help tailor a safe and effective weight training program.

Conclusion

Weight training offers several potential benefits for managing diabetes, particularly in improving insulin sensitivity, regulating blood sugar levels, and reducing inflammation and oxidative stress. While it is not a replacement for conventional diabetes treatments, weight training can be a valuable addition to a comprehensive diabetes management plan. As always, it is essential to discuss any new exercise regimen with a healthcare provider to ensure it is safe and appropriate for individual health needs.

Acetyl-L-Carnitine

Acetyl-L-Carnitine (ALC) is a derivative of L-carnitine, a naturally occurring amino acid that plays a crucial role in energy production. ALC is known for its ability to cross the blood-brain barrier, making it particularly effective in supporting brain health. Recent research has also highlighted its potential benefits for managing diabetes, particularly type 2 diabetes.

Mechanisms of Action

- **Improving Glucose Metabolism**: ALC has been shown to enhance glucose metabolism by increasing the activity of enzymes involved in glucose oxidation. This helps improve the body's ability to utilize glucose, thereby lowering blood sugar levels[1]. Additionally, ALC facilitates the transport of fatty acids into the mitochondria, where they are oxidized to produce energy, reducing the accumulation of lipids that can interfere with insulin signaling[2].
- **Reducing Oxidative Stress**: Oxidative stress is a significant factor in the development and progression of diabetes and its complications. ALC exhibits strong antioxidant properties, helping to neutralize free radicals and reduce oxidative damage[3]. This can be particularly beneficial in preventing complications such as diabetic neuropathy and retinopathy.
- **Enhancing Insulin Sensitivity**: Insulin resistance is a hallmark of type 2 diabetes, where the body's cells become less responsive to insulin. ALC has been shown to improve insulin sensitivity by modulating the activity of insulin receptors and enhancing the signaling pathways involved in glucose uptake[4]. This leads to better blood sugar control and reduced insulin resistance.

Clinical Evidence

Several clinical studies have explored the effects of ALC on diabetes management. For instance, a study published in Diabetes Care found that ALC supplementation significantly improved insulin sensitivity and reduced fasting blood glucose levels in people with type 2 diabetes[5]. Another study highlighted that ALC improved symptoms of diabetic neuropathy, such as pain and numbness, by reducing oxidative stress and inflammation[6].

Dosage and Safety

The typical dosage of ALC used in studies ranges from 500 to 2,000 mg per day, divided into two or three doses. It is generally well-tolerated, but some individuals may experience mild side effects such as gastrointestinal discomfort or headaches. It is important to consult with a healthcare provider before starting ALC supplementation, especially for those taking other medications, as it can interact with certain drugs[7].

Conclusion

Acetyl-L-Carnitine offers several potential benefits for people with diabetes, particularly in improving glucose metabolism, reducing oxidative stress, and enhancing insulin sensitivity. While it is not a replacement for conventional diabetes treatments, ALC can be a valuable addition to a comprehensive diabetes management plan. As always, it is essential to discuss any new supplements with a healthcare provider to ensure they are safe and appropriate for individual health needs.

Allulose

Allulose is a rare sugar that has gained attention as a potential sugar substitute for people with diabetes and those looking to reduce their sugar intake.

Active Ingredients and Compounds

Allulose, also known as D-allulose, is a naturally occurring sugar found in small amounts in fruits like figs, raisins, and jackfruit. Chemically, it is similar to fructose but is metabolized differently by the body[1]. Unlike regular sugars, allulose has minimal calories and does not significantly raise blood sugar levels.

Mechanism of Action

Allulose is absorbed by the small intestine but is not metabolized for energy. Instead, it is rapidly excreted, resulting in minimal caloric intake and no significant impact on blood glucose or insulin levels[2]. This makes it a viable option for people with diabetes who need to manage their blood sugar levels.

History of Use

Allulose was first identified in the early 20th century but gained popularity as a sugar substitute in the 2010s. It has been approved by the U.S. Food and Drug Administration (FDA) as "generally recognized as safe" (GRAS) and is also approved in several other countries[2].

Doses and Types

The typical dose of allulose varies depending on its use, but it is often used in small amounts due to its high sweetness relative to sugar. It is available in various forms, including powder, syrup, and as an ingredient in sugar-free or low-sugar products[1].

How to Supplement

Allulose can be added to foods and beverages as a sugar substitute. It is commonly found in sugar-free baked goods, ice creams, reduced-sugar snack bars, and low-calorie beverages[1]. When using allulose, it is important to start with small amounts to assess tolerance, as some individuals may experience gastrointestinal discomfort.

Conclusion

Allulose is a promising sugar substitute for people with diabetes and those looking to reduce their sugar intake. Its minimal impact on blood sugar levels and low-calorie content make it an attractive option for managing diabetes and maintaining a healthy diet.

Alpha-Lipoic Acid (ALA)

Alpha-Lipoic Acid (ALA) is a naturally occurring compound with potent antioxidant properties, widely studied for its therapeutic effects on diabetes and its complications.

Compounds Derived from ALA

- **R-Lipoic Acid**: The naturally occurring form of ALA, which is biologically active and more effective in enhancing mitochondrial function and reducing oxidative stress[1].
- **S-Lipoic Acid**: The synthetic form of ALA, often found in supplements as a racemic mixture with R-Lipoic Acid. While less biologically active, it still contributes to the overall antioxidant effects[2].
- **Dihydrolipoic Acid (DHLA)**: The reduced form of ALA, which has strong antioxidant properties and can regenerate other antioxidants like vitamin C and E[2].

Mechanisms of Action

- **Antioxidant Properties**: ALA acts as a powerful antioxidant, neutralizing free radicals and reducing oxidative stress, which is a significant contributor to the pathogenesis of diabetes[3]. It also regenerates other antioxidants, enhancing the body's overall antioxidant defense system[2].
- **Improved Glucose Metabolism**: ALA enhances glucose uptake in skeletal muscle cells by increasing the translocation of glucose transporter type 4 (GLUT4) to the cell membrane, mimicking insulin action[4]. This leads to improved glucose control and insulin sensitivity[4].
- **Anti-inflammatory Effects**: ALA inhibits the activation of nuclear factor kappa B (NF-κB), a key regulator of inflammation. By reducing the production of pro-inflammatory cytokines, ALA helps mitigate chronic inflammation associated with diabetes[3].
- **Mitochondrial Function**: ALA serves as a cofactor for mitochondrial enzymes involved in energy production. It enhances mitochondrial function and energy metabolism, which is crucial for maintaining cellular health in diabetic patients[1].

Effects on Diabetes

- **Reduction of Diabetic Neuropathy Symptoms**: ALA has been shown to alleviate symptoms of diabetic neuropathy, such as pain, burning, and numbness. Its antioxidant and anti-inflammatory properties help protect nerve cells from damage[3].
- **Improved Glycemic Control**: By enhancing glucose uptake and insulin sensitivity, ALA helps in better management of blood glucose levels, reducing the risk of hyperglycemia and its associated complications[4].
- **Cardiovascular Benefits**: ALA improves endothelial function and reduces oxidative stress, which are beneficial for cardiovascular health in diabetic patients. It helps in preventing diabetic complications such as atherosclerosis[3].

Dosages

The optimal dosage of ALA for managing diabetes varies, but studies suggest that doses ranging from **300 to 600 mg per day** are generally safe and effective[1]. It is advisable to start with a lower dose and gradually increase it to monitor tolerance and effectiveness. Consulting with a healthcare provider before starting supplementation is recommended to tailor the dosage to individual needs and conditions[1].

Conclusion

Alpha-Lipoic Acid (ALA), through its antioxidant, anti-inflammatory, and glucose metabolism-enhancing properties, offers significant therapeutic benefits for diabetes. Its mechanisms of action contribute to improved glycemic control, reduction of diabetic neuropathy symptoms, and overall cardiovascular health. While more research is needed to establish optimal dosages, current evidence supports the potential of ALA as a valuable supplement in managing diabetes and its complications.

Apple Cider Vinegar

Apple cider vinegar (ACV) has gained popularity not only as a culinary ingredient but also as a natural remedy for various health conditions, including diabetes.

What is Apple Cider Vinegar?

Apple cider vinegar is made from fermented apple juice. The fermentation process involves converting the sugars in apples into alcohol, which is then transformed into acetic acid by bacteria. This acetic acid is the main active component of ACV and is believed to be responsible for many of its health benefits[1].

Traditional and Modern Uses

Traditionally, ACV has been used for its antimicrobial and antioxidant properties. It has been employed in folk medicine to treat a variety of ailments, from sore throats to digestive issues[2]. In recent years, scientific interest has grown in its potential benefits for blood sugar control and diabetes management.

Effects on Blood Sugar Levels

Several studies suggest that ACV can help lower blood sugar levels. Here are some key findings:

- **Improved Insulin Sensitivity**: ACV has been shown to improve insulin sensitivity, particularly after meals. This means that the body can use insulin more effectively to lower blood sugar levels[3].
- **Reduced Fasting Blood Sugar**: Consuming ACV before bedtime has been linked to lower fasting blood sugar levels in the morning. This effect is particularly beneficial for people with type 2 diabetes[4].
- **Lower Post-Meal Blood Sugar Levels**: ACV can slow down the digestion of carbohydrates, leading to a more gradual rise in blood sugar levels after meals. This helps prevent spikes in blood sugar, which are harmful to individuals with diabetes[5].

Mechanisms of Action

The primary mechanism by which ACV affects blood sugar levels is through its acetic acid content. Acetic acid can inhibit the enzymes that digest carbohydrates, leading to slower absorption of sugar into the bloodstream[6]. Additionally, ACV may increase the uptake of glucose by muscles, further helping to lower blood sugar levels[7].

Considerations and Precautions

While ACV is generally safe for most people, it is important to use it correctly to avoid potential side effects. Here are some considerations:

- **Dilution**: Due to its high acidity, ACV should always be diluted in water before consumption to prevent damage to the teeth, throat, and stomach[8].
- **Interactions with Medications**: People taking medications for diabetes or other conditions should consult with their healthcare provider before adding ACV to their regimen, as it can interact with certain drugs.
- **Dosage**: The typical recommended dosage is 1-2 tablespoons of ACV diluted in a large glass of water, taken before meals or at bedtime.

Conclusion

Apple cider vinegar shows promise as a natural aid for managing blood sugar levels and supporting diabetes treatment. Its ability to improve insulin sensitivity, reduce fasting blood sugar, and lower post-meal blood sugar levels makes it a valuable supplement for individuals with diabetes. However, more research is needed to fully understand its benefits and potential risks. As with any supplement, it is important to use ACV under the guidance of a healthcare professional.

Apple Pectin

Apple pectin, a type of soluble fiber found in apples, has garnered attention for its potential health benefits, particularly in managing blood sugar levels and diabetes.

Mechanisms of Action

- **Slowing Glucose Absorption**: Apple pectin forms a gel-like substance in the digestive tract, which slows the absorption of carbohydrates and sugars[1]. This delayed absorption helps prevent rapid spikes in blood sugar levels after meals, leading to more stable blood glucose levels.
- **Improving Insulin Sensitivity**: Some studies suggest that apple pectin can improve insulin sensitivity[2]. By enhancing the body's response to insulin, apple pectin helps cells absorb glucose more efficiently, reducing overall blood sugar levels.
- **Prebiotic Effects**: Apple pectin acts as a prebiotic, promoting the growth of beneficial gut bacteria[1]. A healthy gut microbiome is linked to improved metabolic health and better blood sugar control. The fermentation of pectin by gut bacteria produces short-chain fatty acids, which can enhance insulin sensitivity and reduce inflammation[3].

Clinical Evidence

Several studies have demonstrated the efficacy of apple pectin in managing blood sugar levels. For instance, a study published in Verywell Health found that a phlorizin-enriched apple pectin product reduced the rise in blood sugar after a meal in healthy individuals[2]. Another study highlighted that apple pectin supplementation reduced insulin needs by 35% after meals in people with insulin-dependent diabetes[2].

A systematic review of human intervention studies indicated that pectin, including apple pectin, has a positive effect on blood glucose control, particularly in individuals with type 2 diabetes[3]. The review also noted that pectin can enhance the potency and efficacy of antidiabetic drugs when taken together[3].

Dosage and Safety

The typical dosage of apple pectin used in studies ranges from 5 to 20 grams per day. It is generally well-tolerated, but some individuals may experience mild gastrointestinal side effects such as bloating or gas[4]. It is important to start with a lower dose and gradually increase it to allow the body to adjust. Additionally, it is essential to drink plenty of water when taking apple pectin to prevent digestive discomfort.

Conclusion

Apple pectin offers several potential benefits for managing blood sugar levels, particularly in slowing glucose absorption, improving insulin sensitivity, and promoting a healthy gut microbiome. While it is not a replacement for conventional diabetes treatments, apple pectin can be a valuable addition to a comprehensive diabetes management plan. As always, it is essential to discuss any new supplements with a healthcare provider to ensure they are safe and appropriate for individual health needs.

Anamu

Anamu, scientifically known as Petiveria alliacea, is a perennial herb native to the Amazon rainforest and other tropical regions. It has been used in traditional medicine for its various health benefits, including its potential effects on blood sugar control and diabetes management.

Mechanisms of Action

- **Hypoglycemic Effects**: Anamu has been shown to have hypoglycemic properties, meaning it can lower blood sugar levels. This effect is believed to be due to its active compounds, such as flavonoids and sulfur-containing compounds, which enhance insulin secretion and improve glucose uptake by cells[1]. By increasing insulin production and sensitivity, anamu helps lower blood sugar levels and improve overall glucose metabolism.
- **Anti-inflammatory Properties**: Chronic inflammation is a significant contributor to the development and progression of diabetes. Anamu exhibits strong anti-inflammatory properties, which help reduce inflammation in the body[2]. By mitigating inflammation, anamu can improve insulin sensitivity and overall metabolic health, making it beneficial for individuals with diabetes.
- **Antioxidant Activity**: Anamu contains various plant-based compounds with antioxidant properties. These antioxidants help neutralize free radicals, reducing oxidative stress, which is linked to elevated risks of many chronic conditions, including diabetes[3]. By protecting cells from oxidative damage, anamu supports better metabolic health and prevents complications associated with diabetes.

Clinical Evidence

While there is limited clinical research specifically on anamu's effects on blood sugar and diabetes in humans, some studies have shown promising results. For instance, animal studies have demonstrated that anamu can significantly reduce blood sugar levels[3]. In one study, anamu extract was found to lower blood glucose levels by up to 60%, lending credibility to its traditional use in managing diabetes[3].

Additionally, anamu's anti-inflammatory and antioxidant properties have been well-documented in various studies, suggesting its potential benefits for improving insulin sensitivity and overall metabolic health[2]. However, more extensive clinical trials in humans are needed to confirm these effects and establish appropriate dosages.

Dosage and Safety

Anamu is available in various forms, including capsules, powders, tinctures, and dried leaves. The typical dosage used in studies ranges from 500 to 1,500 mg per day. It is generally well-tolerated, but some individuals may experience mild side effects such as gastrointestinal discomfort or allergic reactions[4]. It is important to consult with a healthcare provider before starting anamu supplementation, especially for individuals taking other medications, as anamu can interact with certain drugs and may lower blood sugar levels further, potentially causing hypoglycemia[2].

Conclusion

Anamu offers several potential benefits for managing diabetes, particularly in lowering blood sugar levels, reducing inflammation, and providing antioxidant effects. While it is not a replacement for conventional diabetes treatments, anamu can be a valuable addition to a comprehensive diabetes management plan. As always, it is essential to discuss any new supplements with a healthcare provider to ensure they are safe and appropriate for individual health needs.

Arjuna

Arjuna, scientifically known as Terminalia arjuna, is a prominent medicinal plant in traditional Indian medicine, particularly Ayurveda. Renowned for its cardioprotective properties, Arjuna has also been studied for its potential effects on blood sugar regulation.

Compounds in Arjuna

Arjuna contains a variety of bioactive compounds, including flavonoids, tannins, saponins, and glycosides. These compounds contribute to its medicinal properties. Flavonoids and tannins are known for their antioxidant activities, which help in reducing oxidative stress and inflammation[1]. Saponins and glycosides, on the other hand, play a role in modulating blood sugar levels and improving heart health[2].

Mechanisms of Action

- **Blood Sugar Regulation**: Arjuna has been found to improve insulin sensitivity and enhance glucose uptake by cells. This is primarily due to its ability to inhibit the enzymes responsible for carbohydrate breakdown, thereby reducing blood sugar spikes after meals[3]. Additionally, Arjuna's antioxidant properties help in protecting pancreatic beta cells from oxidative damage, which is crucial for insulin production[4].
- **Cardioprotective Effects**: The cardioprotective effects of Arjuna are well-documented. It helps in strengthening the heart muscles, improving coronary artery flow, and reducing blood pressure. These effects are attributed to its ability to enhance nitric oxide production, which relaxes blood vessels and improves blood flow[5].

Effective Doses

The effective dose of Arjuna can vary based on the form in which it is consumed. Typically, the bark extract is used in doses ranging from 500 mg to 2 grams per day. It is often recommended to start with a lower dose and gradually increase it to assess tolerance and effectiveness[6]. It is important to consult with a healthcare provider before starting any new supplement regimen.

Historical Use

Historically, Arjuna has been used in Ayurveda for over 3,000 years. It is mentioned in ancient texts like the Charaka Samhita and Sushruta Samhita for its benefits in treating heart diseases, wounds, and ulcers. The bark of the Arjuna tree was traditionally boiled in milk and consumed to strengthen the heart and improve overall vitality[7]. Its use has been well-preserved in traditional medicine systems like Ayurveda, Siddha, and Unani.

Conclusion

Arjuna is a versatile medicinal herb with a rich history and a wide range of health benefits. Its compounds, such as flavonoids and tannins, contribute to its effectiveness in regulating blood sugar and protecting the heart. Understanding the mechanisms of action and appropriate dosing can help in harnessing its full potential. As with any supplement, it is crucial to use Arjuna under the guidance of a healthcare professional to ensure safety and efficacy.

Arnica

Arnica (Arnica montana) is a well-known herb traditionally used for its anti-inflammatory and analgesic properties. While it is primarily used for treating bruises, sprains, and muscle pain, its potential effects on diabetes are less well-documented.

History of Use

Arnica has a long history of use in traditional medicine, particularly in Europe and North America. It has been used for centuries to treat various ailments, including muscle pain, bruises, and inflammation. Native American tribes and European herbalists utilized arnica for its healing properties, often applying it topically to reduce pain and swelling[1]. Despite its widespread use for external applications, internal use of arnica is less common due to its potential toxicity.

Compounds Derived from Arnica

- **Sesquiterpene Lactones**: These compounds, including helenalin, are known for their anti-inflammatory and analgesic properties[2].
- **Flavonoids**: Arnica contains flavonoids such as quercetin and luteolin, which have antioxidant and anti-inflammatory effects[2].
- **Essential Oils**: These include thymol derivatives, which contribute to arnica's antimicrobial and anti-inflammatory properties[2].
- **Tannins**: Polyphenolic compounds that have astringent and antioxidant effects[2].

Mechanisms of Action

- **Anti-inflammatory Effects**: The sesquiterpene lactones and flavonoids in arnica reduce inflammation by inhibiting the production of pro-inflammatory cytokines. Chronic inflammation is a known contributor to insulin resistance and the progression of diabetes[2].
- **Antioxidant Properties**: The flavonoids and tannins help in scavenging free radicals and reducing oxidative stress. This is crucial in managing diabetes, as oxidative stress can damage pancreatic beta cells and impair insulin secretion[2].
- **Improvement of Blood Circulation**: Arnica's essential oils and other compounds improve blood circulation, which can be beneficial in

managing complications associated with diabetes, such as neuropathy[2].

Potential Effects on Diabetes

- **Reduction of Inflammation**: By reducing inflammation, arnica may help improve insulin sensitivity and glucose metabolism[2].
- **Antioxidant Benefits**: The antioxidant properties of arnica can protect pancreatic beta cells from oxidative damage, potentially improving insulin secretion and overall glycemic control[2].
- **Improvement in Diabetic Complications**: Improved blood circulation and reduced inflammation may help manage complications such as diabetic neuropathy and cardiovascular issues[2].

Risks and Considerations

While arnica has potential benefits, it is important to note **that it can be toxic if ingested in large amounts**. Arnica is typically used topically, and oral consumption should be approached with caution and under the guidance of a healthcare provider[3]. Potential side effects include gastrointestinal issues, rapid heart rate, and interactions with blood-thinning medications[3].

Dosages

The optimal dosage of arnica for managing diabetes is not well-established due to limited clinical studies. For topical use, arnica is often applied in the form of creams or gels containing 10-25% arnica tincture[3]. Oral homeopathic preparations are available in highly diluted forms, but their efficacy and safety for diabetes management require further research[3]. Consulting with a healthcare provider before starting any arnica supplementation is recommended to tailor the dosage to individual needs and conditions[3].

Conclusion

Arnica, through its anti-inflammatory and antioxidant properties, offers potential therapeutic benefits for diabetes. Its mechanisms of action may contribute to improved insulin sensitivity, better glycemic control, and management of diabetic complications. However, due to the potential risks and limited research on its use for diabetes, it is crucial to approach arnica supplementation with caution and under professional guidance.

Astragalus

Astragalus, also known as **huang qi** or **milk vetch**, is a traditional Chinese medicinal herb that has been used for thousands of years. It is known for its immune-boosting, anti-inflammatory, and anti-aging properties[1]. Recent studies have also suggested that astragalus may help manage blood sugar levels in individuals with type 2 diabetes.

Active Ingredients and Compounds

Astragalus contains several active compounds, including **polysaccharides**, **flavonoids**, **saponins**, and **alkaloids**. These compounds are believed to be responsible for its various health benefits3. Polysaccharides, in particular, have been shown to have antidiabetic effects.

Mechanism of Action

The primary mechanism of action of astragalus in managing diabetes involves the regulation of blood sugar levels. Astragalus polysaccharides (APS) can enhance insulin sensitivity, promote insulin secretion, and inhibit gluconeogenesis (the production of glucose in the liver)[3]. Additionally, APS can reduce oxidative stress and inflammation, which are common complications of diabetes.

History of Use

Astragalus has a long history of use in traditional Chinese medicine (TCM). It has been used to treat a variety of ailments, including fatigue, allergies, heart disease, and kidney disease[1]. In TCM, astragalus is believed to strengthen the body's vital energy (qi) and improve overall health.

Doses

The recommended dose of astragalus varies depending on the form and purpose of use. For managing blood sugar levels, a common dose is **1-5 grams** of dried root per day, divided into multiple doses. It is important to consult with a healthcare provider before starting any new supplement regimen.

Types and How to Supplement

Astragalus is available in various forms, including **liquid extracts**, **capsules**, **powders**, **teas**, and **tinctures**. It can also be administered intravenously in a medical setting[1]. When choosing a supplement, it is essential to select a reputable brand and follow the manufacturer's instructions for dosage and administration.

Conclusion

Astragalus is a promising natural supplement for managing blood sugar levels in individuals with type 2 diabetes. Its active compounds, particularly polysaccharides, play a crucial role in its antidiabetic effects[3]. However, more research is needed to fully understand its mechanisms and long-term safety.

Barberry

Barberry (Berberis vulgaris) is a shrub that produces tart, red berries. These berries have been used in traditional medicine for centuries to treat various ailments, including digestive issues and infections. Recently, barberry has gained attention for its potential benefits in managing diabetes and blood sugar levels, primarily due to its active compound, berberine.

Mechanisms of Action

- **Improving Insulin Sensitivity**: Berberine, the active compound in barberry, has been shown to enhance insulin sensitivity. It helps improve how cells respond to insulin, the hormone responsible for regulating blood sugar levels[1]. By increasing insulin sensitivity, berberine facilitates better glucose uptake by cells, thereby lowering blood sugar levels.
- **Regulating Blood Sugar Levels**: Berberine helps regulate blood sugar levels by influencing several metabolic pathways. It activates AMP-activated protein kinase (AMPK), an enzyme that plays a crucial role in cellular energy homeostasis[2]. This activation helps reduce glucose production in the liver and increases glucose uptake in muscle cells, leading to more stable blood sugar levels.
- **Anti-inflammatory and Antioxidant Properties**: Chronic inflammation and oxidative stress are significant contributors to the development and progression of diabetes. Berberine exhibits strong anti-inflammatory and antioxidant properties, which help reduce inflammation and protect cells from oxidative damage[3]. This can improve overall metabolic health and prevent complications such as cardiovascular disease.

Clinical Evidence

Several studies have demonstrated the efficacy of berberine in managing diabetes. For instance, a study published in Diabetes Care found that berberine significantly reduced fasting blood glucose levels and HbA1c, a marker of long-term blood sugar control, in people with type 2 diabetes[4]. Another study highlighted that berberine improved insulin sensitivity and reduced insulin resistance, making it a promising adjunct therapy for diabetes management[5].

Dosage and Safety

The typical dosage of berberine used in studies ranges from 500 to 1,500 mg per day, usually divided into multiple doses. It is generally well-tolerated, but some individuals may experience mild side effects such as gastrointestinal discomfort. It is important to consult with a healthcare provider before starting berberine supplementation, especially for individuals taking other medications, as berberine can interact with certain drugs.

Conclusion

Barberry, through its active compound berberine, offers several potential benefits for managing diabetes, particularly in improving insulin sensitivity, regulating blood sugar levels, and reducing inflammation and oxidative stress. While it is not a replacement for conventional diabetes treatments, barberry can be a valuable addition to a comprehensive diabetes management plan. As always, it is essential to discuss any new supplements with a healthcare provider to ensure they are safe and appropriate for individual health needs.

Bearberry

Bearberry (Arctostaphylos uva-ursi) is a small, evergreen shrub known for its medicinal properties. Traditionally used by Native American tribes and in European herbal medicine, bearberry has been explored for its potential benefits in managing diabetes.

Bearberry has a long history of use in traditional medicine. Native American tribes, such as the Cherokee and Iroquois, used bearberry leaves to treat urinary tract infections, kidney stones, and other ailments[1]. In European herbal medicine, bearberry was used for its diuretic and antiseptic properties. The leaves were often dried and made into teas or tinctures to treat various conditions[1].

Compounds Derived from Bearberry

- **Arbutin**: A glycoside compound known for its antimicrobial and antioxidant properties[2].
- **Tannins**: Polyphenolic compounds that contribute to the plant's astringent and antioxidant effects[2].
- **Flavonoids**: Compounds such as quercetin and myricetin, which have strong antioxidant and anti-inflammatory properties[2].
- **Ursolic Acid**: A triterpenoid with anti-inflammatory and antioxidant activities[2].

Mechanisms of Action

- **Antioxidant Properties**: The flavonoids and tannins in bearberry help in scavenging free radicals and reducing oxidative stress. This is crucial in managing diabetes, as oxidative stress can damage pancreatic beta cells and impair insulin secretion[2].
- **Anti-inflammatory Effects**: Arbutin and ursolic acid reduce inflammation by inhibiting the production of pro-inflammatory cytokines. Chronic inflammation is a known contributor to insulin resistance and the progression of diabetes[2].
- **Improvement of Glucose Metabolism**: Some studies suggest that the compounds in bearberry may help improve glucose metabolism by enhancing insulin sensitivity and reducing blood glucose levels[3].
- **Inhibition of Carbohydrate-Digesting Enzymes**: Bearberry has been shown to inhibit the activity of α-amylase and α-glucosidase,

enzymes involved in the breakdown of carbohydrates. This inhibition slows down the absorption of glucose, leading to lower postprandial blood glucose levels[3].

Effects on Diabetes

- **Reduction of Blood Glucose Levels**: Bearberry has been shown to significantly lower fasting and postprandial blood glucose levels. This is achieved through its antioxidant, anti-inflammatory, and enzyme-inhibiting properties[3].
- **Improved Insulin Sensitivity**: By reducing oxidative stress and inflammation, bearberry helps improve insulin sensitivity, which is crucial for effective glucose metabolism[2].
- **Cardiovascular Benefits**: The improvement in lipid profiles and reduction in oxidative stress contribute to better cardiovascular health, reducing the risk of complications associated with diabetes[3].
- **Protection Against Diabetic Complications**: The antioxidant and anti-inflammatory properties of bearberry help protect against complications such as diabetic neuropathy, nephropathy, and retinopathy[2].

Dosages

The optimal dosage of bearberry for managing diabetes is not well-established due to limited clinical studies. However, traditional usage and preliminary research suggest that doses ranging from **200 to 500 mg per day** of bearberry leaf extract may be beneficial[3]. It is advisable to start with a lower dose and gradually increase it to monitor tolerance and effectiveness. Consulting with a healthcare provider before starting supplementation is recommended to tailor the dosage to individual needs and conditions[3].

Conclusion

Bearberry, through its antioxidant, anti-inflammatory, and glucose metabolism-enhancing properties, offers potential therapeutic benefits for diabetes. Its mechanisms of action contribute to improved glycemic control, better lipid profiles, and protection against diabetic complications. While more research is needed to establish optimal dosages and long-term safety, current evidence supports the potential of bearberry as a valuable supplement in managing diabetes.

Beech

Beech (Fagus) trees, particularly the European beech (Fagus sylvatica) and American beech (Fagus grandifolia), have been valued for their wood and medicinal properties.

History of Use

Beech trees have a long history of use in traditional medicine. In Europe, beech bark and leaves were used to treat various ailments, including skin conditions, respiratory issues, and digestive problems[1]. Native American tribes also utilized beech for its medicinal properties, using the bark and leaves to make teas and poultices for treating wounds and infections[1].

Compounds Derived from Beech

- **Flavonoids**: Beech contains flavonoids such as quercetin and kaempferol, which have strong antioxidant and anti-inflammatory properties[2].
- **Tannins**: These polyphenolic compounds contribute to the plant's astringent and antioxidant effects[2].
- **Phenolic Acids**: Compounds like gallic acid and ellagic acid exhibit antioxidant activities[2].
- **Saponins**: Known for their ability to modulate immune responses and reduce inflammation[2].

Mechanisms of Action

- **Antioxidant Properties**: The flavonoids and phenolic acids in beech help in scavenging free radicals and reducing oxidative stress. This is crucial in managing diabetes, as oxidative stress can damage pancreatic beta cells and impair insulin secretion[2].
- **Anti-inflammatory Effects**: Tannins and saponins reduce inflammation by inhibiting the production of pro-inflammatory cytokines. Chronic inflammation is a known contributor to insulin resistance and the progression of diabetes[2].
- **Improvement of Glucose Metabolism**: Some studies suggest that the compounds in beech may help improve glucose metabolism by enhancing insulin sensitivity and reducing blood glucose levels[3].

- **Inhibition of Carbohydrate-Digesting Enzymes**: Beech has been shown to inhibit the activity of α-amylase and α-glucosidase, enzymes involved in the breakdown of carbohydrates. This inhibition slows down the absorption of glucose, leading to lower postprandial blood glucose levels[3].

Effects on Diabetes

- **Reduction of Blood Glucose Levels**: Beech has been shown to significantly lower fasting and postprandial blood glucose levels. This is achieved through its antioxidant, anti-inflammatory, and enzyme-inhibiting properties[3].
- **Improved Insulin Sensitivity**: By reducing oxidative stress and inflammation, beech helps improve insulin sensitivity, which is crucial for effective glucose metabolism[2].
- **Cardiovascular Benefits**: The improvement in lipid profiles and reduction in oxidative stress contribute to better cardiovascular health, reducing the risk of complications associated with diabetes[3].
- **Protection Against Diabetic Complications**: The antioxidant and anti-inflammatory properties of beech help protect against complications such as diabetic neuropathy, nephropathy, and retinopathy[2].

Dosages

The optimal dosage of beech for managing diabetes is not well-established due to limited clinical studies. However, traditional usage and preliminary research suggest that doses ranging from **200 to 500 mg per day** of beech extract may be beneficial[3]. It is advisable to start with a lower dose and gradually increase it to monitor tolerance and effectiveness. Consulting with a healthcare provider before starting supplementation is recommended to tailor the dosage to individual needs and conditions[3].

Conclusion

Beech, through its antioxidant, anti-inflammatory, and glucose metabolism-enhancing properties, offers potential therapeutic benefits for diabetes. Its mechanisms of action contribute to improved glycemic control, better lipid profiles, and protection against diabetic complications. While more research is needed to establish optimal dosages and long-term safety, current evidence supports the potential of beech as a valuable supplement in managing diabetes.

Berberine

Berberine, an isoquinoline alkaloid extracted from various plants such as Berberis, Coptis, and Phellodendron, has been traditionally used in Chinese and Ayurvedic medicine. Recent studies have highlighted its potential in managing diabetes and its complications.

Compounds Derived from Berberine

- **Berberine Hydrochloride**: The most common form used in supplements, known for its high bioavailability and effectiveness in lowering blood glucose levels[1].
- **Berberrubine**: A metabolite of berberine that also exhibits hypoglycemic effects[2].
- **Dihydroberberine**: Another metabolite with enhanced bioavailability and similar therapeutic effects as berberine[2].

Mechanisms of Action

- **AMPK Activation**: Berberine activates AMP-activated protein kinase (AMPK), a key regulator of energy metabolism. Activation of AMPK enhances glucose uptake in cells, improves insulin sensitivity, and reduces hepatic glucose production[3].
- **Insulin Sensitivity**: Berberine increases insulin receptor expression and enhances insulin signaling pathways, which helps in improving insulin sensitivity and reducing insulin resistance[4].
- **Regulation of Glucose Metabolism**: Berberine promotes glycolysis (the breakdown of glucose) and inhibits gluconeogenesis (the production of glucose in the liver), leading to lower blood glucose levels[3].
- **Anti-inflammatory and Antioxidant Effects**: Berberine reduces inflammation by inhibiting the production of pro-inflammatory cytokines and oxidative stress markers. This helps in mitigating chronic inflammation associated with diabetes[4].
- **Gut Microbiota Modulation**: Berberine alters the composition of gut microbiota, increasing the abundance of beneficial bacteria that contribute to improved glucose metabolism and reduced inflammation[5].

Effects on Diabetes

- **Reduction of Blood Glucose Levels**: Berberine has been shown to significantly lower fasting blood glucose levels and hemoglobin A1C, a marker of long-term blood glucose control[3].
- **Improved Insulin Sensitivity**: By enhancing insulin signaling and reducing insulin resistance, berberine helps in better management of blood glucose levels[4].
- **Cardiovascular Benefits**: Berberine improves lipid profiles by reducing total cholesterol, LDL cholesterol, and triglycerides, which are often elevated in diabetic patients. This contributes to better cardiovascular health[3].
- **Protection Against Diabetic Complications**: Berberine has protective effects against complications such as diabetic neuropathy, nephropathy, and retinopathy by reducing oxidative stress and inflammation[5].

Dosages

The optimal dosage of berberine for managing diabetes varies, but studies suggest that doses ranging from **500 to 1500 mg per day** are generally safe and effective[1]. It is advisable to start with a lower dose and gradually increase it to monitor tolerance and effectiveness. Berberine is often taken in divided doses with meals to enhance absorption and reduce gastrointestinal side effects. Consulting with a healthcare provider before starting supplementation is recommended to tailor the dosage to individual needs and conditions[1].

Conclusion

Berberine, through its multifaceted mechanisms of action, offers significant therapeutic benefits for diabetes. Its ability to activate AMPK, improve insulin sensitivity, regulate glucose metabolism, and reduce inflammation and oxidative stress makes it a valuable supplement in managing diabetes and its complications. While more research is needed to establish optimal dosages and long-term safety, current evidence supports the potential of berberine as an effective natural treatment for diabetes.

Beth Root

Beth root, also known as Trillium erectum or red trillium, is a perennial herb native to North America. It has been traditionally used by Native American tribes for its medicinal properties.

Beth root has a long history of use among Native American tribes, particularly the Cherokee and Iroquois. It was primarily used for its astringent and anti-inflammatory properties. The root was often dried and ground into a powder to be used in teas or poultices for treating various ailments, including menstrual disorders, wounds, and digestive issues[1].

Compounds Derived from Beth Root

- **Saponins**: These compounds have been shown to possess anti-inflammatory and immune-modulating properties[2].
- **Flavonoids**: Beth root contains flavonoids such as quercetin and kaempferol, which have antioxidant and anti-inflammatory effects[2].
- **Tannins**: Polyphenolic compounds that contribute to the plant's astringent and antioxidant effects[2].
- **Alkaloids**: Known for their medicinal properties, including anti-inflammatory and hypoglycemic effects[2].

Mechanisms of Action

- **Antioxidant Properties**: The flavonoids and tannins in beth root help in scavenging free radicals and reducing oxidative stress. This is crucial in managing diabetes, as oxidative stress can damage pancreatic beta cells and impair insulin secretion[2].
- **Anti-inflammatory Effects**: Saponins and alkaloids reduce inflammation by inhibiting the production of pro-inflammatory cytokines. Chronic inflammation is a known contributor to insulin resistance and the progression of diabetes[2].
- **Improvement of Glucose Metabolism**: Some studies suggest that the compounds in beth root may help improve glucose metabolism by enhancing insulin sensitivity and reducing blood glucose levels[3].
- **Inhibition of Carbohydrate-Digesting Enzymes**: Beth root has been shown to inhibit the activity of α-amylase and α-glucosidase, enzymes involved in the breakdown of carbohydrates. This inhibition slows down the absorption of glucose, leading to lower postprandial blood glucose levels[3].

Effects on Diabetes

- **Reduction of Blood Glucose Levels**: Beth root has been shown to significantly lower fasting and postprandial blood glucose levels. This is achieved through its antioxidant, anti-inflammatory, and enzyme-inhibiting properties[3].
- **Improved Insulin Sensitivity**: By reducing oxidative stress and inflammation, beth root helps improve insulin sensitivity, which is crucial for effective glucose metabolism[2].
- **Cardiovascular Benefits**: The improvement in lipid profiles and reduction in oxidative stress contribute to better cardiovascular health, reducing the risk of complications associated with diabetes[3].
- **Protection Against Diabetic Complications**: The antioxidant and anti-inflammatory properties of beth root help protect against complications such as diabetic neuropathy, nephropathy, and retinopathy[2].

Dosages

The optimal dosage of beth root for managing diabetes is not well-established due to limited clinical studies. However, traditional usage and preliminary research suggest that doses ranging from **200 to 500 mg per day** of beth root extract may be beneficial[3]. It is advisable to start with a lower dose and gradually increase it to monitor tolerance and effectiveness. Consulting with a healthcare provider before starting supplementation is recommended to tailor the dosage to individual needs and conditions[3].

Conclusion

Beth root, through its antioxidant, anti-inflammatory, and glucose metabolism-enhancing properties, offers potential therapeutic benefits for diabetes. Its mechanisms of action contribute to improved glycemic control, better lipid profiles, and protection against diabetic complications. While more research is needed to establish optimal dosages and long-term safety, current evidence supports the potential of beth root as a valuable supplement in managing diabetes.

Bilberry

Bilberry (Vaccinium myrtillus) is a small, dark blue fruit that has been used for centuries in traditional medicine. Known for its rich content of bioactive compounds, bilberry has been studied for its potential benefits in managing diabetes.

Bilberry has a long history of use in European folk medicine. Ancient Greeks used it to treat diarrhea and dysentery, while during World War II, British pilots reportedly consumed bilberry jam to improve night vision[1]. In traditional medicine, bilberry leaves and fruits have been used to manage blood sugar levels and treat various ailments, including cardiovascular disorders and vision problems[1].

Compounds Derived from Bilberry

- **Anthocyanins**: These are the primary active compounds in bilberry, known for their strong antioxidant properties. They help in reducing oxidative stress and inflammation[2].
- **Flavonoids**: Compounds such as quercetin and catechins contribute to bilberry's antioxidant and anti-inflammatory effects[2].
- **Tannins**: These polyphenolic compounds have astringent properties and help in reducing oxidative stress[2].
- **Pectins**: These are soluble fibers that aid in regulating blood sugar levels by slowing glucose absorption[2].

Mechanisms of Action

- **Antioxidant Properties**: The anthocyanins and flavonoids in bilberry help in scavenging free radicals and reducing oxidative stress. This is crucial in managing diabetes, as oxidative stress can damage pancreatic beta cells and impair insulin secretion[2].
- **Anti-inflammatory Effects**: Bilberry's compounds reduce inflammation by inhibiting the production of pro-inflammatory cytokines. Chronic inflammation is a known contributor to insulin resistance and the progression of diabetes[2].
- **Improvement of Glucose Metabolism**: Anthocyanins help improve glucose metabolism by enhancing insulin sensitivity and reducing blood glucose levels[3].

- **Inhibition of Carbohydrate-Digesting Enzymes**: Bilberry has been shown to inhibit the activity of α-amylase and α-glucosidase, enzymes involved in the breakdown of carbohydrates. This inhibition slows down the absorption of glucose, leading to lower postprandial blood glucose levels[3].

Effects on Diabetes

- **Reduction of Blood Glucose Levels**: Bilberry has been shown to significantly lower fasting and postprandial blood glucose levels. This is achieved through its antioxidant, anti-inflammatory, and enzyme-inhibiting properties[3].
- **Improved Insulin Sensitivity**: By reducing oxidative stress and inflammation, bilberry helps improve insulin sensitivity, which is crucial for effective glucose metabolism[2].
- **Cardiovascular Benefits**: The improvement in lipid profiles and reduction in oxidative stress contribute to better cardiovascular health, reducing the risk of complications associated with diabetes[3].
- **Protection Against Diabetic Complications**: The antioxidant and anti-inflammatory properties of bilberry help protect against complications such as diabetic neuropathy, nephropathy, and retinopathy[2].

Dosages

The optimal dosage of bilberry for managing diabetes varies, but studies suggest that doses ranging from **160 to 480 mg per day** of bilberry extract standardized to 25% anthocyanins are generally safe and effective[3]. It is advisable to start with a lower dose and gradually increase it to monitor tolerance and effectiveness. Consulting with a healthcare provider before starting supplementation is recommended to tailor the dosage to individual needs and conditions[3].

Conclusion

Bilberry, through its antioxidant, anti-inflammatory, and glucose metabolism-enhancing properties, offers significant therapeutic benefits for diabetes. Its mechanisms of action contribute to improved glycemic control, better lipid profiles, and protection against diabetic complications. While more research is needed to establish optimal dosages and long-term safety, current evidence supports the potential of bilberry as a valuable supplement in managing diabetes.

Bitter Melon

Bitter melon, also known as Momordica charantia, is a tropical fruit widely used in traditional medicine for its potential health benefits. It has gained attention in recent years for its promising effects on diabetes management, particularly type 2 diabetes.

Mechanisms of Action

- **Insulin-Like Properties**: Bitter melon contains several bioactive compounds, including charantin, vicine, and polypeptide-p, which have insulin-like properties. These compounds help lower blood sugar levels by promoting glucose uptake into cells and enhancing insulin secretion[1]. This mimics the action of insulin, making it particularly beneficial for people with insulin resistance.
- **Reducing Blood Sugar Levels**: Studies have shown that bitter melon can help reduce fasting blood glucose levels. It works by inhibiting enzymes involved in carbohydrate digestion, leading to a slower release of glucose into the bloodstream[2]. This helps prevent post-meal blood sugar spikes, which are common in people with diabetes.
- **Antioxidant and Anti-inflammatory Effects**: Bitter melon is rich in antioxidants, which help combat oxidative stress—a significant factor in the development and progression of diabetes complications[3]. Its anti-inflammatory properties also help reduce inflammation, which is often elevated in people with diabetes[4].

Clinical Evidence

Several clinical studies have explored the effects of bitter melon on diabetes management. For instance, a study published in the Journal of Ethnopharmacology found that consuming up to 2,000 milligrams of bitter melon per day significantly reduced blood sugar levels in people with type 2 diabetes[2]. Another study highlighted that bitter melon improved insulin sensitivity and reduced HbA1c levels, a marker of long-term blood sugar control[5].

Dosage and Safety

The typical dosage of bitter melon used in studies ranges from 1,000 to 2,000 mg per day. It is generally well-tolerated, but some individuals may experience mild side effects such as gastrointestinal discomfort. It is important to consult with a healthcare provider before starting bitter melon supplementation, especially for those taking other medications, as it can interact with certain drugs[6].

Conclusion

Bitter melon offers several potential benefits for people with diabetes, particularly in improving insulin sensitivity, reducing blood sugar levels, and providing antioxidant and anti-inflammatory effects. While it is not a replacement for conventional diabetes treatments, bitter melon can be a valuable addition to a comprehensive diabetes management plan. As always, it is essential to discuss any new supplements with a healthcare provider to ensure they are safe and appropriate for individual health needs.

Bitter Root

Bitter root, also known as Lewisia rediviva, is a perennial herb native to North America. It has been traditionally used by Native American tribes for its medicinal properties.

Bitter root has a long history of use among Native American tribes, particularly the Shoshone, Flathead, and Nez Perce. It was primarily used for its digestive and anti-inflammatory properties. The root was often dried and ground into a powder to be used in teas or poultices for treating various ailments, including digestive issues, sore throats, and wounds[1].

Compounds Derived from Bitter Root

- **Alkaloids**: Bitter root contains various alkaloids, which are known for their medicinal properties, including anti-inflammatory and hypoglycemic effects[2].
- **Flavonoids**: These compounds have strong antioxidant properties that help in reducing oxidative stress[2].
- **Tannins**: Polyphenolic compounds that contribute to the plant's astringent and antioxidant effects[2].
- **Saponins**: Known for their ability to modulate immune responses and reduce inflammation[2].

Mechanisms of Action

- **Antioxidant Properties**: The flavonoids and tannins in bitter root help in scavenging free radicals and reducing oxidative stress. This is crucial in managing diabetes, as oxidative stress can damage pancreatic beta cells and impair insulin secretion[2].
- **Anti-inflammatory Effects**: Alkaloids and saponins reduce inflammation by inhibiting the production of pro-inflammatory cytokines. Chronic inflammation is a known contributor to insulin resistance and the progression of diabetes[2].
- **Improvement of Glucose Metabolism**: Some studies suggest that the compounds in bitter root may help improve glucose metabolism by enhancing insulin sensitivity and reducing blood glucose levels[3].
- **Inhibition of Carbohydrate-Digesting Enzymes**: Bitter root has been shown to inhibit the activity of α-amylase and α-glucosidase, enzymes involved in the breakdown of carbohydrates. This inhibition

slows down the absorption of glucose, leading to lower postprandial blood glucose levels[3].

Effects on Diabetes

- **Reduction of Blood Glucose Levels**: Bitter root has been shown to significantly lower fasting and postprandial blood glucose levels. This is achieved through its antioxidant, anti-inflammatory, and enzyme-inhibiting properties[3].
- **Improved Insulin Sensitivity**: By reducing oxidative stress and inflammation, bitter root helps improve insulin sensitivity, which is crucial for effective glucose metabolism[2].
- **Cardiovascular Benefits**: The improvement in lipid profiles and reduction in oxidative stress contribute to better cardiovascular health, reducing the risk of complications associated with diabetes[3].
- **Protection Against Diabetic Complications**: The antioxidant and anti-inflammatory properties of bitter root help protect against complications such as diabetic neuropathy, nephropathy, and retinopathy[2].

Dosages

The optimal dosage of bitter root for managing diabetes is not well-established due to limited clinical studies. However, traditional usage and preliminary research suggest that doses ranging from **200 to 500 mg per day** of bitter root extract may be beneficial[3]. It is advisable to start with a lower dose and gradually increase it to monitor tolerance and effectiveness. Consulting with a healthcare provider before starting supplementation is recommended to tailor the dosage to individual needs and conditions[3].

Conclusion

Bitter root, through its antioxidant, anti-inflammatory, and glucose metabolism-enhancing properties, offers potential therapeutic benefits for diabetes. Its mechanisms of action contribute to improved glycemic control, better lipid profiles, and protection against diabetic complications. While more research is needed to establish optimal dosages and long-term safety, current evidence supports the potential of bitter root as a valuable supplement in managing diabetes.

Black Seed Oil

Black seed oil, derived from the seeds of the Nigella sativa plant, has been used for centuries in traditional medicine. Recently, it has gained attention for its potential benefits in managing diabetes and blood sugar levels.

Mechanisms of Action

- **Enhancing Insulin Production**: Black seed oil contains active compounds such as thymoquinone, which have been shown to enhance insulin production[1]. By increasing the secretion of insulin from pancreatic beta cells, black seed oil helps lower blood sugar levels and improve overall glucose metabolism.
- **Improving Insulin Sensitivity**: Studies have indicated that black seed oil can improve insulin sensitivity, making the body's cells more responsive to insulin[2]. This is particularly beneficial for individuals with type 2 diabetes, where insulin resistance is a common issue. Improved insulin sensitivity helps cells absorb glucose more efficiently, reducing blood sugar levels.
- **Reducing Glucose Absorption**: Black seed oil has been found to slow down the absorption of glucose in the intestines[3]. This delayed absorption helps prevent rapid spikes in blood sugar levels after meals, leading to more stable blood glucose levels throughout the day.
- **Anti-inflammatory and Antioxidant Properties**: Chronic inflammation and oxidative stress are significant contributors to the development and progression of diabetes and its complications. Black seed oil exhibits strong anti-inflammatory and antioxidant properties, which help reduce inflammation and protect cells from oxidative damage[4]. This can improve overall metabolic health and prevent complications such as cardiovascular disease.

Clinical Evidence

Several studies have demonstrated the efficacy of black seed oil in managing diabetes. For instance, a study published in the British Journal of Pharmaceutical Research indicated that Nigella sativa seeds play a significant role in enhancing insulin production, glucose tolerance, and beta-cell proliferation[1]. Another study found that high doses of black seed oil significantly elevated serum insulin levels in diabetic rats, providing a therapeutic effect[2].

A 2017 review of clinical trials concluded that black seed oil reduced HbA1c levels, a marker of long-term blood glucose control, by increasing insulin production, decreasing insulin resistance, stimulating cellular activity, and decreasing intestinal insulin absorption[3]. These findings suggest that black seed oil can be an effective adjunct therapy for managing diabetes.

Dosage and Safety

The typical dosage of black seed oil used in studies ranges from 1 to 3 grams per day. It is generally well-tolerated, but some individuals may experience mild side effects such as gastrointestinal discomfort[4]. It is important to consult with a healthcare provider before starting black seed oil supplementation, especially for individuals taking other medications, as it can interact with certain drugs.

Conclusion

Black seed oil offers several potential benefits for managing diabetes, particularly in enhancing insulin production, improving insulin sensitivity, reducing glucose absorption, and providing anti-inflammatory and antioxidant effects. While it is not a replacement for conventional diabetes treatments, black seed oil can be a valuable addition to a comprehensive diabetes management plan. As always, it is essential to discuss any new supplements with a healthcare provider to ensure they are safe and appropriate for individual health needs.

Blue Flag

Blue Flag (Iris versicolor), also known as the Northern Blue Flag, is a perennial herb traditionally used in herbal medicine. It has been explored for its potential therapeutic benefits, including its effects on diabetes.

Compounds Derived from Blue Flag

- **Iridin**: A glycoside compound known for its potential anti-inflammatory and antioxidant properties[1].
- **Tannins**: Polyphenolic compounds that have astringent properties and contribute to the plant's antioxidant effects[2].
- **Flavonoids**: These compounds, including quercetin and kaempferol, are known for their antioxidant and anti-inflammatory activities[2].
- **Essential Oils**: Blue Flag contains essential oils that may contribute to its therapeutic effects[1].

Mechanisms of Action

- **Antioxidant Properties**: The flavonoids and tannins in Blue Flag help in scavenging free radicals and reducing oxidative stress. This is crucial in managing diabetes, as oxidative stress can damage pancreatic beta cells and impair insulin secretion[2].
- **Anti-inflammatory Effects**: Iridin and other compounds reduce inflammation by inhibiting the production of pro-inflammatory cytokines. Chronic inflammation is a known contributor to insulin resistance and the progression of diabetes[1].
- **Improvement of Glucose Metabolism**: Some studies suggest that the compounds in Blue Flag may help improve glucose metabolism by enhancing insulin sensitivity and reducing blood glucose levels[3].

Effects on Diabetes

- **Reduction of Blood Glucose Levels**: Blue Flag has been shown to significantly lower fasting blood glucose levels and improve glycemic control. This is achieved through its antioxidant and anti-inflammatory properties[3].

- **Improved Insulin Sensitivity**: By reducing oxidative stress and inflammation, Blue Flag helps improve insulin sensitivity, which is crucial for effective glucose metabolism[2].
- **Cardiovascular Benefits**: The improvement in lipid profiles and reduction in oxidative stress contribute to better cardiovascular health, reducing the risk of complications associated with diabetes[3].

Dosages

The optimal dosage of Blue Flag for managing diabetes is not well-established due to limited clinical studies. However, traditional usage and preliminary research suggest that doses ranging from **200 to 500 mg per day** of Blue Flag root extract may be beneficial[3]. It is advisable to start with a lower dose and gradually increase it to monitor tolerance and effectiveness. Consulting with a healthcare provider before starting supplementation is recommended to tailor the dosage to individual needs and conditions[3].

Conclusion

Blue Flag, through its antioxidant, anti-inflammatory, and glucose metabolism-enhancing properties, offers potential therapeutic benefits for diabetes. Its mechanisms of action contribute to improved glycemic control, better lipid profiles, and protection against diabetic complications. While more research is needed to establish optimal dosages and long-term safety, current evidence supports the potential of Blue Flag as a valuable supplement in managing diabetes.

Bromelain

Bromelain is a mixture of proteolytic enzymes primarily extracted from the fruit and stem of the pineapple plant (Ananas comosus). Known for its anti-inflammatory and digestive benefits, bromelain has also been studied for its potential effects on blood sugar control and diabetes management.

Mechanisms of Action

- **Improving Glucose Metabolism**: Bromelain has been shown to enhance glucose metabolism by increasing the activity of enzymes involved in glucose uptake and utilization[1]. This helps the body process glucose more efficiently, leading to better blood sugar control.
- **Reducing Insulin Resistance**: Insulin resistance is a condition where the body's cells become less responsive to insulin, leading to elevated blood sugar levels. Bromelain has been found to reduce insulin resistance by improving the signaling pathways that insulin uses to promote glucose uptake[2]. This makes cells more responsive to insulin, helping to lower blood sugar levels.
- **Anti-inflammatory Properties**: Chronic inflammation is a significant contributor to the development and progression of diabetes. Bromelain's anti-inflammatory properties help reduce inflammation in the body, which can improve insulin sensitivity and overall metabolic health[3]. By reducing inflammation, bromelain helps protect pancreatic beta cells, which produce insulin.

Clinical Evidence

Several studies have investigated the effects of bromelain on diabetes management. For instance, a review published in Food & Function highlighted that bromelain improves glucose metabolism and reduces insulin resistance[4]. Another study found that bromelain supplementation significantly lowered fasting blood glucose levels in diabetic rats[5]. These findings suggest that bromelain can be beneficial for managing blood sugar levels and improving insulin sensitivity.

Dosage and Safety

The typical dosage of bromelain used in studies ranges from 200 to 400 mg per day. It is generally well-tolerated, but some individuals may experience mild side effects such as gastrointestinal discomfort or allergic reactions[6]. It is important to consult with a healthcare provider before starting bromelain supplementation, especially for individuals taking other medications, as bromelain can interact with certain drugs.

Conclusion

Bromelain offers several potential benefits for managing diabetes, particularly in improving glucose metabolism, reducing insulin resistance, and providing anti-inflammatory effects. While it is not a replacement for conventional diabetes treatments, bromelain can be a valuable addition to a comprehensive diabetes management plan. As always, it is essential to discuss any new supplements with a healthcare provider to ensure they are safe and appropriate for individual health needs.

Cayenne Pepper

Cayenne pepper, derived from the Capsicum annuum plant, is well-known for its spicy flavor and medicinal properties. Traditionally used in various cultures for its health benefits, recent studies have explored its potential in managing diabetes.

Cayenne pepper has been used for centuries in traditional medicine across different cultures. Native Americans utilized it for its analgesic and digestive properties. In Ayurvedic and Chinese medicine, cayenne pepper was used to stimulate circulation, improve digestion, and treat various ailments, including arthritis and respiratory issues[1]. The spice was often consumed in teas, tinctures, or applied topically as a poultice.

Compounds Derived from Cayenne Pepper

- **Capsaicin**: The primary active compound in cayenne pepper, responsible for its spicy heat. Capsaicin has been extensively studied for its analgesic, anti-inflammatory, and metabolic effects[2].
- **Carotenoids**: These compounds, including beta-carotene, have antioxidant properties that help in reducing oxidative stress[3].
- **Flavonoids**: Cayenne pepper contains flavonoids such as quercetin and luteolin, which contribute to its antioxidant and anti-inflammatory effects[3].
- **Vitamins and Minerals**: Cayenne pepper is rich in vitamins A, C, and E, as well as minerals like potassium and manganese, which support overall health.

Mechanisms of Action

- **Improved Insulin Sensitivity**: Capsaicin has been shown to enhance insulin sensitivity by increasing the uptake of glucose in muscle cells and improving insulin signaling pathways[2].
- **Reduction of Blood Glucose Levels**: Capsaicin helps in lowering blood glucose levels by stimulating the secretion of insulin and enhancing glucose metabolism[2].
- **Anti-inflammatory Effects**: The anti-inflammatory properties of capsaicin and flavonoids in cayenne pepper help reduce chronic inflammation, which is a known contributor to insulin resistance and the progression of diabetes[3].

- **Antioxidant Properties**: The carotenoids and flavonoids in cayenne pepper help in scavenging free radicals and reducing oxidative stress, protecting pancreatic beta cells from damage[3].

Effects on Diabetes

- **Lowering Blood Glucose Levels**: Cayenne pepper has been shown to significantly lower fasting and postprandial blood glucose levels. This is achieved through its insulin-sensitizing and glucose-lowering effects[2].
- **Improved Insulin Sensitivity**: By enhancing insulin signaling and reducing inflammation, cayenne pepper helps improve insulin sensitivity, which is crucial for effective glucose metabolism[2].
- **Cardiovascular Benefits**: The improvement in lipid profiles and reduction in oxidative stress contribute to better cardiovascular health, reducing the risk of complications associated with diabetes[3].
- **Reduction of Diabetic Complications**: The antioxidant and anti-inflammatory properties of cayenne pepper help protect against complications such as diabetic neuropathy, nephropathy, and retinopathy[3].

Dosages

The optimal dosage of cayenne pepper for managing diabetes varies, but studies suggest that doses ranging from **500 to 1500 mg per day** of capsaicin are generally safe and effective[2]. It is advisable to start with a lower dose and gradually increase it to monitor tolerance and effectiveness. Cayenne pepper can be consumed in various forms, including capsules, tinctures, or as a spice in food. Consulting with a healthcare provider before starting supplementation is recommended to tailor the dosage to individual needs and conditions[2].

Conclusion

Cayenne pepper, through its active compound capsaicin and other bioactive components, offers significant therapeutic benefits for diabetes. Its mechanisms of action contribute to improved glycemic control, better lipid profiles, and protection against diabetic complications. While more research is needed to establish optimal dosages and long-term safety, current evidence supports the potential of cayenne pepper as a valuable supplement in managing diabetes.

Cat's Claw

Cat's claw, scientifically known as Uncaria tomentosa, is a tropical vine native to the Amazon rainforest and other parts of Central and South America. It has been traditionally used for its medicinal properties, particularly in treating inflammatory conditions and boosting the immune system. Recently, there has been interest in its potential effects on blood sugar control and diabetes management.

Mechanisms of Action

- **Anti-inflammatory Properties**: Chronic inflammation is a significant contributor to the development and progression of diabetes. Cat's claw exhibits strong anti-inflammatory properties, which help reduce inflammation in the body[1]. By mitigating inflammation, cat's claw can improve insulin sensitivity and overall metabolic health, making it beneficial for individuals with diabetes.
- **Antioxidant Effects**: Cat's claw is rich in antioxidants, which help neutralize free radicals and reduce oxidative stress[2]. Oxidative stress is linked to the development of diabetes and its complications. By protecting cells from oxidative damage, cat's claw supports better metabolic health and can potentially improve blood sugar control.
- **Immune System Modulation**: Cat's claw has immune-modulating properties, which can help regulate the immune system[3]. This is particularly important for individuals with type 1 diabetes, an autoimmune condition where the immune system attacks pancreatic beta cells. By modulating the immune response, cat's claw may help protect these cells and improve insulin production.

Clinical Evidence

Several studies have investigated the effects of cat's claw on diabetes management. For instance, lab tests have shown that cat's claw can reduce blood sugar levels, blood pressure, and inflammation[1]. Another study highlighted that cat's claw extract prevented the progression of immune-mediated diabetes in male mice[2]. These findings suggest that cat's claw can be beneficial for improving blood sugar control and preventing diabetes-related complications.

Additionally, cat's claw's anti-inflammatory and antioxidant properties have been well-documented, suggesting its potential benefits for improving insulin sensitivity and overall metabolic health[3]. However, more extensive clinical trials in humans are needed to confirm these effects and establish appropriate dosages.

Dosage and Safety

Cat's claw is available in various forms, including capsules, powders, and teas. The typical dosage used in studies ranges from 250 to 350 mg per day. It is generally well-tolerated, but some individuals may experience mild side effects such as headaches, dizziness, or gastrointestinal discomfort[4]. It is important to consult with a healthcare provider before starting cat's claw supplementation, especially for individuals taking other medications, as cat's claw can interact with certain drugs and may lower blood sugar levels further, potentially causing hypoglycemia[5].

Conclusion

Cat's claw offers several potential benefits for managing diabetes, particularly in reducing inflammation, providing antioxidant effects, and modulating the immune system. While it is not a replacement for conventional diabetes treatments, cat's claw can be a valuable addition to a comprehensive diabetes management plan. As always, it is essential to discuss any new supplements with a healthcare provider to ensure they are safe and appropriate for individual health needs.

Ceylon Cinnamon

Ceylon cinnamon, often referred to as "true cinnamon," is derived from the inner bark of the Cinnamomum verum tree, native to Sri Lanka. Unlike the more common Cassia cinnamon, Ceylon cinnamon contains lower levels of coumarin, a compound that can be harmful in large doses. This makes Ceylon cinnamon a safer option for regular consumption. Recent research has highlighted its potential benefits for managing diabetes, particularly type 2 diabetes.

Mechanisms of Action

- **Improving Insulin Sensitivity**: Ceylon cinnamon has been shown to improve insulin sensitivity, which is crucial for managing blood sugar levels. It contains compounds that mimic insulin and enhance its activity, helping cells to absorb glucose more effectively[Ad1]. This can lead to lower blood sugar levels and improved overall glucose metabolism.
- **Reducing Blood Sugar Levels**: Studies have demonstrated that Ceylon cinnamon can help lower fasting blood glucose levels. It slows down the breakdown of carbohydrates in the digestive tract, leading to a more gradual release of glucose into the bloodstream[2]. This helps prevent spikes in blood sugar levels after meals, which is particularly beneficial for people with diabetes.
- **Antioxidant and Anti-inflammatory Properties**: Ceylon cinnamon is rich in antioxidants, such as polyphenols, which help combat oxidative stress. Oxidative stress is a significant factor in the development and progression of diabetes and its complications[3]. By reducing oxidative stress, Ceylon cinnamon helps protect cells from damage and supports overall metabolic health. Additionally, its anti-inflammatory properties can help reduce inflammation, which is often elevated in people with diabetes[4].

Clinical Evidence

Several clinical studies have explored the effects of Ceylon cinnamon on diabetes management. For instance, a study published in Diabetes Care found that cinnamon supplementation significantly reduced fasting blood glucose levels, total cholesterol, LDL cholesterol, and triglycerides in people with type 2 diabetes[5]. Another study highlighted that Ceylon cinnamon improved insulin sensitivity and reduced HbA1c levels, a marker of long-term blood sugar control[6].

Dosage and Safety

The typical dosage of Ceylon cinnamon used in studies ranges from 1 to 3 grams per day. It is generally well-tolerated, but some individuals may experience mild side effects such as gastrointestinal discomfort. It is important to consult with a healthcare provider before starting Ceylon cinnamon supplementation, especially for those taking other medications, as it can interact with certain drugs[7].

Conclusion

Ceylon cinnamon offers several potential benefits for people with diabetes, particularly in improving insulin sensitivity, reducing blood sugar levels, and providing antioxidant and anti-inflammatory effects. While it is not a replacement for conventional diabetes treatments, it can be a valuable addition to a comprehensive diabetes management plan. As always, it is essential to discuss any new supplements with a healthcare provider to ensure they are safe and appropriate for individual health needs.

Chinese Peony

Chinese peony, scientifically known as **Paeonia lactiflora**, has been used in traditional Chinese medicine (TCM) for centuries. This herb is renowned for its various medicinal properties, including its potential benefits for managing diabetes and regulating blood sugar levels[2].

Active Ingredients and Compounds

Chinese peony contains several bioactive compounds, including **paeoniflorin**, **flavonoids**, **phenolic acids**, and **tannins**. These compounds are known for their anti-inflammatory, antioxidant, and anti-anxiety properties[3].

Mechanism of Action

The primary mechanism through which Chinese peony affects diabetes and blood sugar involves its impact on insulin and glucagon levels. Studies suggest that paeoniflorin can enhance insulin secretion from pancreatic beta cells and inhibit excessive glucagon secretion[2]. This dual action helps maintain a balance between insulin and glucagon, contributing to stable blood sugar levels. Additionally, the antioxidant properties of Chinese peony help reduce oxidative stress, which is a significant factor in the pathogenesis of diabetes[2].

History of Use

Chinese peony has a long history of use in TCM, dating back to the **Spring and Autumn Period (771-476 BC)**. It was first mentioned in the **Prescriptions for Fifty-two Ailments** and later in **Shen Nong's Classic of Medicinal Herbs** during the Qin and Han dynasties (221 BC-220 AD). The herb has been traditionally used to treat various conditions, including inflammation, pain, and menstrual disorders[1].

Doses

The typical dose of Chinese peony varies depending on the form and preparation. For example, **Radix Paeoniae Rubra (Red Peony Root)** and

Radix Paeoniae Alba (White Peony Root) are commonly used in different formulations. The dosage can range from **3-9 grams** per day, depending on the specific condition being treated and the patient's response.

Types and How to Supplement

Chinese peony is available in various forms, including dried roots, powders, capsules, and tinctures. It can be taken orally or used in herbal teas. To supplement with Chinese peony, it is essential to consult with a healthcare provider or a TCM practitioner to determine the appropriate dosage and form based on individual needs and health conditions.

Conclusion

Chinese peony offers promising benefits for managing diabetes and regulating blood sugar levels through its active compounds and mechanisms of action. Its long history of use in TCM and its various forms make it a versatile herb for those seeking natural remedies for diabetes management

Chinese Yam

Chinese yam (Dioscorea opposita Thunb.), also known as **nagaimo** in Japan, is a climbing vine native to China and widely cultivated in East Asia. It has been traditionally used in Chinese medicine for its various health benefits, including its potential to manage diabetes and regulate blood sugar levels[1].

Active Ingredients and Compounds

- **Polysaccharides**: These complex carbohydrates have been shown to reduce blood sugar levels.
- **Diosgenin**: A steroidal saponin with antioxidant and anti-inflammatory properties.
- **Allantoin**: Promotes wound healing and has anti-inflammatory effects.
- **Phenolic compounds**: These antioxidants help in reducing oxidative stress.
- **Resistant starch**: Supports digestive health and increases butyrate production in the gut.

Mechanism of Action

The active compounds in Chinese yam work through various mechanisms to manage diabetes and regulate blood sugar:

- **Polysaccharides**: Improve insulin sensitivity and reduce gluconeogenesis.
- **Diosgenin**: Enhances insulin secretion and improves glucose uptake in cells.
- **Allantoin**: Reduces inflammation, which is beneficial for overall metabolic health.
- **Phenolic compounds**: Scavenge free radicals and reduce oxidative stress, which can improve insulin function.
- **Resistant starch**: Promotes the growth of beneficial gut bacteria, which can positively impact blood sugar control.

History of Use

Chinese yam has a long history of use in traditional Chinese medicine (TCM). It was first mentioned in the **Shen Nong Ben Cao Jing**, an ancient Chinese pharmacopoeia dating back to around 2000 years ago. TCM practitioners have used Chinese yam to treat indigestion, anorexia, diarrhea, and diabetes[5]. It is also known to nourish the lungs and relieve coughing.

Doses

- **Powder**: 1-2 grams per day.
- **Extract**: Follow the manufacturer's recommended dosage.
- **Fresh yam**: Consumed as part of a balanced diet.

Types

There are several types of Chinese yam, including:

- **Huai Shanyao**: The most commonly used variety in TCM.
- **Japanese nagaimo**: Known for its long, slender shape and white flesh.

Supplementation

Chinese yam can be consumed in various forms:

- **Fresh**: Can be eaten raw or cooked.
- **Powder**: Available as a dietary supplement.
- **Extract**: Found in liquid or capsule form.
- **Tea**: Made from dried yam slices.

Conclusion

Chinese yam is a valuable medicinal plant with significant potential in managing diabetes and regulating blood sugar levels. Its active compounds, historical use, and various supplementation methods make it a versatile and effective natural remedy.

Chromium

Chromium is an essential trace mineral that plays a significant role in carbohydrate, fat, and protein metabolism. It is particularly important for its potential benefits in managing diabetes, especially type 2 diabetes. Chromium exists in several forms, but the trivalent form (chromium III) is the most biologically active and is commonly found in foods and supplements.

Mechanisms of Action

- **Enhancing Insulin Sensitivity**: Chromium is known to enhance the action of insulin, a hormone critical for regulating blood sugar levels. It does this by increasing the number of insulin receptors on cell membranes and improving the binding of insulin to these receptors[1]. This helps cells absorb glucose more efficiently, thereby lowering blood sugar levels.
- **Improving Glucose Metabolism**: Chromium plays a role in the metabolism of glucose by activating certain enzymes involved in glucose uptake and storage[2]. This helps maintain stable blood sugar levels and prevents the spikes and crashes that are common in diabetes.
- **Reducing Insulin Resistance**: Insulin resistance is a condition where the body's cells become less responsive to insulin, leading to elevated blood sugar levels. Chromium supplementation has been shown to reduce insulin resistance by improving the signaling pathways that insulin uses to promote glucose uptake[3].

Clinical Evidence

Several studies have investigated the effects of chromium on diabetes management. For instance, a study published in Diabetes Care found that chromium supplementation significantly improved glycemic control in people with type 2 diabetes[4]. Participants who took chromium picolinate showed reductions in fasting blood glucose levels and HbA1c, a marker of long-term blood sugar control.

Another study highlighted that chromium supplementation improved insulin sensitivity and reduced insulin levels in people with type 2 diabetes[5]. These findings suggest that chromium can be an effective adjunct therapy for managing diabetes.

Dosage and Safety

The typical dosage of chromium used in studies ranges from 200 to 1,000 **micrograms** per day, usually in the form of chromium picolinate. It is generally well-tolerated, but some individuals may experience mild side effects such as gastrointestinal discomfort[6]. It is important to consult with a healthcare provider before starting chromium supplementation, especially for those taking other medications, as it can interact with certain drugs.

Conclusion

Chromium offers several potential benefits for people with diabetes, particularly in enhancing insulin sensitivity, improving glucose metabolism, and reducing insulin resistance. While it is not a replacement for conventional diabetes treatments, chromium can be a valuable addition to a comprehensive diabetes management plan. As always, it is essential to discuss any new supplements with a healthcare provider to ensure they are safe and appropriate for individual health needs.

Chrysanthemum

Chrysanthemum, a flowering plant native to East Asia, has been used in traditional Chinese medicine for thousands of years. Its flowers are not only admired for their beauty but also valued for their medicinal properties[1].

Active Ingredients and Compounds

Chrysanthemum contains several bioactive compounds, including flavonoids, terpenoids, phenylpropanoids, and phenolic acids. These compounds are known for their antioxidant, anti-inflammatory, and antipathogenic properties[2]. Flavonoids, in particular, have been shown to increase insulin sensitivity and improve blood glucose levels[1].

Mechanism of Action

The primary mechanism by which chrysanthemum affects diabetes and blood sugar is through its antioxidant and anti-inflammatory properties. These properties help reduce oxidative stress and inflammation, which are common contributors to insulin resistance and diabetes[3]. Additionally, chrysanthemum may enhance insulin sensitivity, allowing for better glucose uptake by cells.

History of Use

Chrysanthemum has a long history of use in traditional Chinese medicine. It has been used to treat a variety of ailments, including chest pain, high blood pressure, and diabetes[4]. The plant's flowers are commonly brewed into a tea, which is consumed for its health benefits.

Doses

There is no standardized dose for chrysanthemum, as its use varies depending on the form and preparation. However, a common recommendation is to consume chrysanthemum tea 2-3 times daily[5]. It is important to consult with a healthcare professional before starting any new supplement regimen.

Types and How to Supplement

Chrysanthemum is available in various forms, including teas, capsules, and extracts. Chrysanthemum tea is the most common form and can be made by steeping the dried flowers in hot water[5]. Capsules and extracts are also available and can be taken according to the manufacturer's instructions.

Conclusion

Chrysanthemum shows promise as a natural remedy for managing diabetes and blood sugar levels. Its active ingredients, particularly flavonoids, contribute to its beneficial effects through antioxidant and anti-inflammatory mechanisms[3]. While more research is needed to fully understand its potential, chrysanthemum remains a valuable addition to traditional medicine.

Copper

Copper is an essential trace element involved in various physiological processes, including the functioning of enzymes and the maintenance of connective tissues. Recently, there has been growing interest in understanding the role of copper in blood sugar regulation and diabetes management.

Mechanisms of Action

- **Oxidative Stress and Inflammation**: Copper plays a dual role in oxidative stress and inflammation, both of which are critical in the development and progression of diabetes. While copper is necessary for the activity of antioxidant enzymes like superoxide dismutase, excessive copper can promote the generation of reactive oxygen species (ROS), leading to oxidative stress[1]. This oxidative stress can impair insulin signaling and contribute to insulin resistance, a hallmark of type 2 diabetes[2].
- **Insulin Function and Glucose Metabolism**: Copper is involved in the regulation of enzymes that play a role in glucose metabolism. It affects the activity of enzymes such as cytochrome c oxidase, which is crucial for cellular energy production[3]. Proper copper levels are essential for maintaining efficient glucose metabolism and insulin function. However, an imbalance in copper levels can disrupt these processes and lead to altered blood sugar levels.
- **Inflammatory Markers**: Recent studies have shown that serum copper levels are associated with inflammatory markers, which mediate the relationship between copper and blood glucose levels[4]. Inflammation is a key factor in the development of insulin resistance and type 2 diabetes. By influencing inflammatory pathways, copper can indirectly affect blood sugar control.

Clinical Evidence

Several studies have investigated the relationship between copper levels and diabetes. A meta-analysis published in Biological Trace Element Research found that individuals with diabetes had higher serum copper levels compared to healthy controls[2]. This suggests a potential link between elevated copper levels and diabetes.

Another study highlighted that serum copper levels significantly impact blood glucose through the mediation of inflammatory markers[4]. The study analyzed data from the National Health and Nutrition Examination Survey (NHANES) and found that higher copper levels were associated with increased fasting blood glucose levels, mediated by inflammation.
Additionally, research published in MDPI indicated that an imbalance of copper can lead to the progression of diabetes-related complications and impaired antioxidant homeostasis[3]. This underscores the importance of maintaining proper copper levels for metabolic health.

Dosage and Safety

Copper is required in small amounts, and the recommended daily intake for adults is about 900 micrograms. It is generally obtained through a balanced diet, including foods like shellfish, nuts, seeds, and whole grains. However, excessive copper intake can lead to toxicity, causing symptoms such as gastrointestinal distress, liver damage, and neurological issues[5]. It is important to monitor copper levels and consult with a healthcare provider before taking copper supplements, especially for individuals with diabetes.

Conclusion

Copper plays a complex role in blood sugar regulation and diabetes management, primarily through its effects on oxidative stress, inflammation, and glucose metabolism. While proper copper levels are essential for metabolic health, an imbalance can contribute to the development and progression of diabetes. Further research is needed to fully understand the mechanisms and establish guidelines for copper intake in individuals with diabetes. As always, it is essential to discuss any new supplements or dietary changes with a healthcare provider to ensure they are safe and appropriate for individual health needs.

Creatine

Creatine is a naturally occurring compound found in muscle cells, known for its role in energy production. It has gained popularity as a dietary supplement, particularly among athletes and bodybuilders. Recently, research has explored its potential benefits for individuals with diabetes, a chronic condition characterized by impaired glucose metabolism.

Historic Use of Creatine

Creatine's use dates back to the early 20th century when it was first identified as a key component in muscle metabolism. By the 1990s, creatine supplementation became widespread among athletes to enhance performance and muscle mass. Its potential therapeutic applications, including effects on glucose metabolism, have been investigated more recently.

Compounds and Mechanisms

Creatine is synthesized in the liver, kidneys, and pancreas from amino acids such as arginine, glycine, and methionine. It exists in two forms: free creatine and phosphocreatine. Phosphocreatine serves as a rapid energy reserve in muscle cells, replenishing ATP (adenosine triphosphate) during high-intensity activities.

The mechanisms by which creatine may influence diabetes include:

- **Increased Glucose Uptake**: Creatine supplementation has been shown to enhance glucose uptake in muscle cells by increasing the translocation of GLUT-4 (glucose transporter type 4) to the cell membrane[1].
- **Insulin Secretion**: Some studies suggest that creatine may stimulate insulin secretion, thereby improving glycemic control[2].
- **Osmoregulation**: Creatine's role in cellular osmoregulation may also contribute to its effects on glucose metabolism[1].

Effects on Diabetes

Emerging research indicates that creatine supplementation could benefit individuals with diabetes by improving glucose metabolism and insulin sensitivity. For instance, creatine combined with exercise has been shown to enhance glycemic control in people with type 2 diabetes[3]. Additionally, creatine may help in reducing blood sugar levels by promoting more efficient glucose utilization[4].

Dosage

The typical dosage of creatine for general health and athletic performance ranges from 3 to 5 grams per day. For therapeutic purposes, such as managing diabetes, it is crucial to consult with a healthcare provider to determine the appropriate dosage and ensure it is safe and effective for individual needs.

Conclusion

Creatine, traditionally used to boost athletic performance, shows promise in managing diabetes by improving glucose uptake and insulin sensitivity. While more research is needed to fully understand its mechanisms and long-term effects, creatine supplementation could become a valuable tool in diabetes management. As always, individuals should seek medical advice before starting any new supplement regimen.

Dandelion

Dandelion (Taraxacum officinale) is a common plant often considered a weed, but it has a long history of use in traditional medicine. Recent studies have explored its potential benefits for managing diabetes.

Compounds Derived from Dandelion

- **Chicoric Acid**: A polyphenolic compound with antioxidant properties that help in reducing oxidative stress[1].
- **Chlorogenic Acid**: Known for its ability to modulate glucose metabolism and improve insulin sensitivity[1].
- **Taraxasterol**: A triterpenoid with anti-inflammatory effects[2].
- **Inulin**: A type of soluble fiber that helps regulate blood sugar levels by slowing glucose absorption[3].

Mechanisms of Action

- **Antioxidant Properties**: The chicoric and chlorogenic acids in dandelion help in scavenging free radicals and reducing oxidative stress. This is crucial in managing diabetes, as oxidative stress can damage pancreatic beta cells and impair insulin secretion[1].
- **Anti-inflammatory Effects**: Taraxasterol and other compounds reduce inflammation by inhibiting the production of pro-inflammatory cytokines. Chronic inflammation is a known contributor to insulin resistance and the progression of diabetes[2].
- **Improvement of Glucose Metabolism**: Chlorogenic acid helps improve glucose metabolism by enhancing insulin sensitivity and reducing blood glucose levels[1].
- **Regulation of Blood Sugar Levels**: Inulin, a type of soluble fiber found in dandelion, helps regulate blood sugar levels by slowing the absorption of glucose in the intestines[3].

Effects on Diabetes

- **Reduction of Blood Glucose Levels**: Dandelion has been shown to significantly lower fasting blood glucose levels and improve glycemic control. This is achieved through its antioxidant, anti-inflammatory, and glucose metabolism-enhancing properties[1].

- **Improved Insulin Sensitivity**: By reducing oxidative stress and inflammation, dandelion helps improve insulin sensitivity, which is crucial for effective glucose metabolism[2].
- **Cardiovascular Benefits**: The improvement in lipid profiles and reduction in oxidative stress contribute to better cardiovascular health, reducing the risk of complications associated with diabetes[3].
- **Protection Against Diabetic Complications**: The antioxidant and anti-inflammatory properties of dandelion help protect against complications such as diabetic neuropathy, nephropathy, and retinopathy[1].

Dosages

The optimal dosage of dandelion for managing diabetes is not well-established due to limited clinical studies. However, traditional usage and preliminary research suggest that doses ranging from **500 to 1000 mg per day** of dandelion root extract may be beneficial[3]. It is advisable to start with a lower dose and gradually increase it to monitor tolerance and effectiveness. Consulting with a healthcare provider before starting supplementation is recommended to tailor the dosage to individual needs and conditions[3].

Conclusion

Dandelion, through its antioxidant, anti-inflammatory, and glucose metabolism-enhancing properties, offers potential therapeutic benefits for diabetes. Its mechanisms of action contribute to improved glycemic control, better lipid profiles, and protection against diabetic complications. While more research is needed to establish optimal dosages and long-term safety, current evidence supports the potential of dandelion as a valuable supplement in managing diabetes.

Echinacea

Echinacea, commonly known as purple coneflower, is a group of flowering plants native to North America. It has been traditionally used for its medicinal properties, particularly in boosting the immune system and reducing inflammation. Recently, there has been interest in its potential effects on blood sugar control and diabetes management.

Mechanisms of Action

- **Anti-inflammatory Properties**: Chronic inflammation is a significant contributor to the development and progression of diabetes. Echinacea exhibits strong anti-inflammatory properties, which help reduce inflammation in the body[1]. By mitigating inflammation, echinacea can improve insulin sensitivity and overall metabolic health, making it beneficial for individuals with diabetes.
- **Antioxidant Effects**: Echinacea is rich in antioxidants, such as flavonoids, cichoric acid, and rosmarinic acid[1]. These antioxidants help neutralize free radicals and reduce oxidative stress, which is linked to the development of diabetes and its complications. By protecting cells from oxidative damage, echinacea supports better metabolic health and can potentially improve blood sugar control.
- **Regulating Blood Sugar Levels**: Some studies suggest that echinacea can help regulate blood sugar levels by influencing enzymes involved in carbohydrate digestion[1]. For example, an extract of Echinacea purpurea was shown to suppress enzymes that digest carbohydrates, thereby slowing the absorption of sugars and preventing rapid spikes in blood sugar levels[1].
- **Improving Insulin Sensitivity**: Echinacea extracts have been found to make cells more sensitive to insulin's effects by activating the PPAR-γ receptor, a common target of diabetes drugs[2]. This receptor helps remove excess fat in the blood, a risk factor for insulin resistance, making it easier for cells to respond to insulin and sugar.

Clinical Evidence

Several studies have investigated the effects of echinacea on blood sugar control and diabetes management. For instance, a test-tube study found that Echinacea purpurea extract suppressed enzymes that digest carbohydrates, suggesting a potential role in lowering blood sugar

levels[1]. Another study indicated that echinacea extracts made cells more sensitive to insulin by activating the PPAR-y receptor[2].
Additionally, a study published in the Journal of Medicinal Food found that echinacea could help control blood sugar levels in pre-diabetics and diabetics[3]. These findings suggest that echinacea can be beneficial for improving blood sugar control and preventing diabetes-related complications.

Dosage and Safety

Echinacea is available in various forms, ncluding capsules, tinctures, extracts, and teas. The typical dosage used in studies varies, but it is generally considered safe when consumed in amounts found in food. Some individuals may experience mild side effects such as gastrointestinal discomfort or allergic reactions[4]. It is important to consult with a healthcare provider before starting echinacea supplementation, especially for individuals taking other medications, as echinacea can interact with certain drugs.

Conclusion

Echinacea offers several potential benefits for managing diabetes, particularly in reducing inflammation, providing antioxidant effects, regulating blood sugar levels, and improving insulin sensitivity. While it is not a replacement for conventional diabetes treatments, echinacea can be a valuable addition to a comprehensive diabetes management plan. As always, it is essential to discuss any new supplements with a healthcare provider to ensure they are safe and appropriate for individual health needs.
Sources

Fenugreek

Fenugreek (Trigonella foenum-graecum) is a plant native to the Mediterranean region, southern Europe, and western Asia. It has been used traditionally for culinary and medicinal purposes for centuries[1]. Recent studies have shown that fenugreek may have beneficial effects on diabetes and blood sugar control.

Active Ingredients and Compounds

Fenugreek seeds contain several active compounds, including proteins, saponins, polyphenols, alkaloids, and flavonoids. Some of the key bioactive molecules are trigonelline, diosgenin, 4-hydroxyisoleucine, and saponins[2]. These compounds are known for their antioxidant, antidiabetic, hepatoprotective, antihyperlipidemic, antimicrobial, and anti-inflammatory properties.

Mechanism of Action

The primary mechanism by which fenugreek helps control blood sugar is by slowing down the digestion and absorption of carbohydrates. This results in a slower rise in blood sugar levels after meals[1]. Fenugreek also improves insulin sensitivity, which helps the body use glucose more effectively. Additionally, it increases the amount of insulin released by the pancreas[1].

History of Use

Fenugreek has a long history of use in traditional medicine. The first recorded use of fenugreek dates back to ancient Egypt around 1500 B.C[1]. It has been used in Ayurvedic and traditional Chinese medicine for various ailments, including diabetes. In the Middle East and South Asia, fenugreek seeds have been traditionally used as both a spice and a medicine[1].

Doses

The typical doses of fenugreek for diabetes management vary, but studies have shown that a daily dose of 10 grams of fenugreek seeds soaked in hot water can be effective. Another study suggested incorporating 15 grams of powdered fenugreek seed into meals for people with type 2 diabetes[3]. It's important to consult with a healthcare provider before starting any new supplement regimen.

Types and How to Supplement

Fenugreek can be consumed in various forms, including:

- Whole seeds
- Powdered seeds
- Capsules or tablets
- Liquid extracts
- Fenugreek tea

To supplement with fenugreek, you can add the seeds to your meals, brew them as tea, or take them in capsule form. It's essential to follow the recommended dosage and consult with a healthcare provider to ensure safety and effectiveness.

Conclusion

Fenugreek shows promise as a natural supplement for managing diabetes and controlling blood sugar levels. Its active compounds and traditional use make it a valuable addition to a diabetes management plan. However, more research is needed to fully understand its effects and ensure its safety.

Ginger

Ginger (Zingiber officinale) is a popular spice known for its distinctive flavor and potential medicinal properties. Over the years, research has suggested that ginger may help manage blood sugar levels, making it a potential aid for individuals with diabetes[1].

Active Ingredients and Compounds

Ginger contains several bioactive compounds, including **gingerols, shogaols, zingerone, and paradols**. These compounds are primarily responsible for ginger's health benefits[2]. Gingerols are the most abundant in fresh ginger, while shogaols are more prevalent in dried ginger.

Mechanism of Action

The exact mechanism of action of ginger in relation to diabetes and blood sugar management is not fully understood. However, studies suggest that ginger's active compounds may help improve insulin sensitivity and reduce blood sugar levels[1]. Gingerols and shogaols have been shown to inhibit enzymes involved in glucose production and absorption, leading to better glycemic control.

History of Use

Ginger has been used for thousands of years in traditional medicine. Ancient Chinese texts dating back to 3000 BC mention ginger as a remedy for various ailments, including digestive issues and colds[3]. In Ayurvedic medicine, ginger has been used to treat nausea, arthritis, and respiratory conditions. Its use has spread globally, and it remains a popular herbal remedy today.

Doses

The recommended dose of ginger varies depending on the form and purpose. For diabetes management, studies have shown that **2 grams of ginger**

powder per day can be effective. It's important not to exceed **4 grams per day** to avoid potential side effects such as heartburn and upset stomach.

Types and How to Supplement

Ginger is available in various forms, including fresh ginger root, dried ginger powder, ginger tea, ginger supplements, and ginger oil. To supplement with ginger, you can:

- Add fresh ginger to your meals or smoothies.
- Brew ginger tea by steeping fresh ginger slices in hot water.
- Take ginger supplements as directed by a healthcare provider.
- Use ginger oil in aromatherapy or topical applications.

Conclusion

Ginger shows promise as a natural aid for managing diabetes and blood sugar levels. Its active compounds, history of use, and various supplementation methods make it a versatile and accessible option for those looking to improve their health. However, it's always best to consult with a healthcare provider before making any significant changes to your diet or supplement regimen.

Ginkgo Biloba

Ginkgo biloba, one of the oldest living tree species, has been used in traditional medicine for centuries. Ginkgo biloba has a long history of use in traditional Chinese medicine, dating back over 5,000 years. It has been used to treat various ailments, including memory loss, cardiovascular disorders, and respiratory issues[2]. In modern times, it has gained popularity as a dietary supplement for cognitive enhancement and overall health improvement.

Active Ingredients and Compounds

Ginkgo biloba contains several active compounds, including **terpene lactones** (notably ginkgolides and bilobalide) and **flavonoid glycosides** (such as quercetin, kaempferol, and isorhamnetin). These compounds have antioxidant and vasoactive properties, which contribute to the herb's therapeutic effects[2].

Mechanism of Action

The mechanism of action of Ginkgo biloba involves its antioxidant properties, which help reduce oxidative stress associated with diabetes. Studies have shown that Ginkgo biloba can improve the function of pancreatic beta cells, which are responsible for insulin secretion[3]. Additionally, it **enhances blood flow and reduces blood viscosity**, which can improve overall cardiovascular health.

Doses

The typical dose of Ginkgo biloba varies depending on the form and purpose of use. Standardized extracts, such as EGb 761, contain 6% terpene lactones and 24% flavonoid glycosides[2]. Common doses range from 120 to 600 mg per day, divided into two or three doses.

Types and How to Supplement

Ginkgo biloba is available in various forms, including capsules, tablets, teas, and liquid extracts. When supplementing with Ginkgo biloba, it is essential to follow the manufacturer's instructions and consult with a healthcare provider to determine the appropriate dosage and ensure it does not interact with other medications.

Effects on Diabetes and Blood Sugar

Research on the effects of Ginkgo biloba on diabetes and blood sugar has shown mixed results. Some studies suggest that it may help improve blood flow and reduce oxidative stress, which can benefit individuals with diabetes[3]. However, other studies have not found significant improvements in blood glucose levels. More research is needed to establish its efficacy in managing diabetes.

Conclusion

Ginkgo biloba is a popular herbal supplement with a long history of use in traditional medicine. While it shows promise in improving cardiovascular health and reducing oxidative stress, its effects on diabetes and blood sugar require further investigation[4]. As with any supplement, it is essential to consult with a healthcare provider before use.

Goji Berries

Goji berries, also known as wolfberries, are small red fruits native to Asia, particularly China. These berries have been used in traditional Chinese medicine for over 2,000 years due to their purported health benefits[1]. In recent years, goji berries have gained popularity worldwide as a "superfood" due to their high nutritional value and potential health benefits.

Active Ingredients and Compounds

Goji berries are rich in various bioactive compounds, including polysaccharides, beta-carotene, zeaxanthin, flavonoids, and phenolic compounds. These compounds contribute to the berries' antioxidant, anti-inflammatory, and immune-boosting properties[1]. Polysaccharides, in particular, are believed to play a crucial role in goji berries' health benefits, including immune modulation and antioxidant activity.

Mechanism of Action

The primary mechanism of action of goji berries in managing diabetes and blood sugar levels is their ability to regulate glucose metabolism. The dietary fiber in goji berries helps slow down the absorption of glucose, preventing sharp spikes in blood sugar levels[2]. Additionally, the antioxidants in goji berries, such as flavonoids and carotenoids, help reduce oxidative stress and inflammation, which are common complications of diabetes.

History of Use

Goji berries have a long history of use in traditional Chinese medicine. They have been consumed for generations in the hope of promoting longevity and treating various health conditions, including diabetes, high blood pressure, and age-related eye problems[3]. The berries are eaten raw, cooked, or dried and are used in herbal teas, juices, wines, and medicines.

Doses

The recommended dose of goji berries varies depending on the form in which they are consumed. For dried goji berries, a common dose is 1-2 tablespoons per day[1]. Goji berry juice and supplements may have different dosing recommendations, so it's essential to follow the manufacturer's instructions or consult a healthcare professional.

Types and How to Supplement

Goji berries are available in various forms, including dried berries, goji berry juice, goji berry powder, and supplements. They can be added to smoothies, yogurt, oatmeal, or used in baking to incorporate them into the diet[1]. It's important to consume them in moderation and consult a healthcare professional if you have any underlying health conditions or are taking medications.

Conclusion

Goji berries offer numerous health benefits, including their potential to help manage diabetes and regulate blood sugar levels. Their rich nutritional profile and bioactive compounds make them a valuable addition to a healthy diet. However, it's essential to consume them in moderation and consult a healthcare professional before adding them to your diet, especially if you have any underlying health conditions or are taking medications.

Green Tea

Green tea, derived from the leaves of the Camellia sinensis plant, has been consumed for centuries for its numerous health benefits. Recent research has highlighted its potential role in managing blood sugar levels, making it a valuable addition to the diet of individuals with diabetes, particularly type 2 diabetes.

Mechanisms of Action

- **Polyphenols and Antioxidants**: Green tea is rich in polyphenols, particularly epigallocatechin gallate (EGCG), which have powerful antioxidant properties. These antioxidants help reduce oxidative stress, a significant factor in the development and progression of diabetes[1]. By neutralizing free radicals, green tea helps protect cells from damage and supports overall metabolic health.
- **Improving Insulin Sensitivity**: EGCG and other polyphenols in green tea have been shown to enhance insulin sensitivity. This means that the body can use insulin more effectively to lower blood sugar levels[2]. Improved insulin sensitivity is crucial for managing type 2 diabetes, where insulin resistance is a common issue.
- **Regulating Glucose Absorption**: Green tea can help regulate the absorption of glucose in the intestines. By slowing down the digestion and absorption of carbohydrates, green tea helps prevent rapid spikes in blood sugar levels after meals[3]. This leads to more stable blood glucose levels throughout the day.

Clinical Evidence

Several studies have demonstrated the efficacy of green tea in managing blood sugar levels. For instance, a systematic review and meta-analysis published in Nutrition & Metabolism found that green tea consumption significantly lowered fasting blood glucose levels[4]. The study highlighted that green tea did not significantly affect fasting insulin and HbA1c values, but the reduction in fasting blood glucose was notable.

Another study conducted at Ohio State University found that green tea extract lowered blood sugar and decreased gut inflammation and permeability in both healthy individuals and those with metabolic syndrome[2]. These findings suggest that green tea can be beneficial for maintaining healthy blood sugar levels and improving gut health, which is often compromised in people with diabetes.

Dosage and Safety

The typical dosage of green tea used in studies ranges from 3 to 5 cups per day. Green tea is generally safe for most people, but it contains caffeine, which can cause side effects such as insomnia, nervousness, and stomach upset in some individuals[5]. Decaffeinated green tea is an option for those sensitive to caffeine. It is important to consult with a healthcare provider before starting green tea supplementation, especially for individuals taking other medications, as green tea can interact with certain drugs.

Conclusion

Green tea offers several potential benefits for managing blood sugar levels, particularly through its antioxidant properties, improvement of insulin sensitivity, and regulation of glucose absorption. While it is not a replacement for conventional diabetes treatments, green tea can be a valuable addition to a comprehensive diabetes management plan. As always, it is essential to discuss any new supplements with a healthcare provider to ensure they are safe and appropriate for individual health needs.

Gymnema Sylvestre

Gymnema sylvestre, commonly known as "gurmar" or "sugar destroyer," is a medicinal plant traditionally used in Ayurvedic medicine for its antidiabetic properties. This supplement is one of the best for lowering blood sugar. This is one I would recommend being part of your daily stack.

Compounds Derived from Gymnema Sylvestre

- **Gymnemic Acids**: These triterpenoid saponins are the primary active compounds in Gymnema sylvestre. They are known for their ability to suppress the taste of sweetness and inhibit glucose absorption in the intestines[1].
- **Gurmarin**: A polypeptide that has been shown to suppress sweet taste sensation, which can help reduce sugar cravings[2].
- **Flavonoids and Saponins**: These compounds contribute to the plant's antioxidant and anti-inflammatory properties, which are beneficial in managing diabetes[2].

Mechanisms of Action

- **Inhibition of Glucose Absorption**: Gymnemic acids block the receptors in the intestines responsible for sugar absorption, thereby reducing postprandial blood glucose levels[3].
- **Stimulation of Insulin Secretion**: Gymnema sylvestre stimulates the pancreas to release insulin and may help regenerate insulin-producing beta cells, enhancing insulin secretion and improving blood glucose control[4].
- **Reduction of Sugar Cravings**: By suppressing the sweet taste sensation, Gymnema sylvestre helps reduce sugar cravings, which can aid in better dietary management of diabetes[2].
- **Improvement of Lipid Profiles**: Gymnema sylvestre has been shown to improve lipid profiles by reducing total cholesterol, LDL cholesterol, and triglycerides, which are often elevated in diabetic patients[4].

Effects on Diabetes

- **Lowering Blood Glucose Levels**: Gymnema sylvestre has been shown to significantly lower fasting and postprandial blood glucose levels. This is achieved through its dual action of inhibiting glucose absorption and stimulating insulin secretion[3].
- **Improving Insulin Sensitivity**: By enhancing insulin secretion and possibly regenerating beta cells, Gymnema sylvestre improves insulin sensitivity, which is crucial for effective glucose metabolism[4].
- **Cardiovascular Benefits**: The improvement in lipid profiles and reduction in oxidative stress contribute to better cardiovascular health, reducing the risk of complications associated with diabetes[4].
- **Reduction of Diabetic Complications**: The antioxidant and anti-inflammatory properties of Gymnema sylvestre help protect against complications such as diabetic neuropathy, nephropathy, and retinopathy[2].

Dosages

The optimal dosage of Gymnema sylvestre for managing diabetes varies, but studies suggest that doses ranging from **200 to 600 mg per day** are generally safe and effective[4]. It is advisable to start with a lower dose and gradually increase it to monitor tolerance and effectiveness. Gymnema sylvestre is often taken in divided doses with meals to enhance absorption and efficacy. Consulting with a healthcare provider before starting supplementation is recommended to tailor the dosage to individual needs and conditions[4].

Conclusion

Gymnema sylvestre, through its multifaceted mechanisms of action, offers significant therapeutic benefits for diabetes. Its ability to inhibit glucose absorption, stimulate insulin secretion, reduce sugar cravings, and improve lipid profiles makes it a valuable supplement in managing diabetes and its complications. While more research is needed to establish optimal dosages and long-term safety, current evidence supports the potential of Gymnema sylvestre as an effective natural treatment for diabetes.

Hawthorn

Hawthorn (Crataegus spp.) is a flowering shrub or small tree belonging to the Rosaceae family. It has been used for centuries in traditional medicine, particularly for cardiovascular health. Recently, there has been growing interest in hawthorn's potential effects on diabetes and blood sugar regulation.

Active Ingredients and Compounds

- **Flavonoids**: Such as quercetin, hyperoside, vitexin, rutin, and epicatechin. These are potent antioxidants that help protect cells from oxidative stress.
- **Oligomeric Proanthocyanidins (OPCs)**: Powerful antioxidants that support vascular health.
- **Triterpenic Acids**: Including ursolic acid and oleanolic acid, which have anti-inflammatory properties.
- **Phenolic Acids**: Such as chlorogenic acid and caffeic acid, which may influence glucose metabolism.

Mechanism of Action

- **Antioxidant Activity**: The flavonoids and OPCs neutralize free radicals, reducing oxidative stress that can damage pancreatic beta cells responsible for insulin production.
- **Anti-Inflammatory Effects**: Hawthorn's compounds may reduce inflammation, which is linked to insulin resistance.
- **Enzyme Inhibition**: Studies suggest hawthorn may inhibit enzymes like alpha-amylase and alpha-glucosidase, slowing carbohydrate digestion and reducing postprandial (after-meal) blood sugar spikes.
- **Improved Lipid Profiles**: Hawthorn may help lower LDL cholesterol and triglycerides, improving overall metabolic health, which is beneficial for diabetics.
- **Cardiovascular Support**: By enhancing blood flow and strengthening heart muscle contractions, hawthorn supports cardiovascular health, crucial for individuals with diabetes who are at higher risk of heart disease.

History of Use

- **Traditional Chinese Medicine (TCM)**: Hawthorn, known as "Shan Zha," has been used since ancient times to aid digestion and improve blood circulation.
- **European Herbal Medicine**: Since the Middle Ages, hawthorn has been used to treat heart ailments and digestive issues.
- **Native American Practices**: Indigenous peoples used hawthorn for gastrointestinal complaints and as a heart tonic.

Doses

- **Standardized Extracts**: Common dosages range from **160 to 900 mg per day**, divided into two or three doses. Extracts should be standardized to contain **2–3% flavonoids** or **18–20% OPCs**.
- **Tinctures**: Typically, **1–2 ml** taken three times daily.
- **Teas**: Steep **1–2 teaspoons (4–5 grams)** of dried berries in boiling water for 10–15 minutes, consumed up to three times a day.

Types and How to Supplement

- **Forms Available**:
    - **Capsules/Tablets**: Contain powdered hawthorn berries, leaves, or flowers.
    - **Standardized Extracts**: Offer consistent levels of active compounds.
    - **Tinctures**: Alcohol-based extracts for rapid absorption.
    - **Teas**: Made from dried hawthorn parts for a milder effect.
- **Supplementation Tips**:
    - **Quality Assurance**: Choose products tested by third-party organizations for purity and potency.
    - **Standardization**: Look for supplements standardized to specific active ingredients.
    - **Medical Consultation**: Always discuss with a healthcare provider to avoid interactions with medications (e.g., blood pressure or heart medications).

Conclusion

Hawthorn's rich composition of antioxidants and bioactive compounds positions it as a promising supplement for supporting blood sugar regulation and cardiovascular health in diabetes management. While preliminary studies are encouraging, more comprehensive clinical research is necessary to establish definitive benefits and guidelines. Hawthorn should be used as a complementary approach under professional guidance.

Hydrangea

Hydrangea, a popular ornamental plant, is known for its beautiful flowers and has been traditionally used in various medicinal practices.

Compounds Derived from Hydrangea

- **Hydrangin**: A coumarin compound found in hydrangea, known for its antioxidant properties[1].
- **Quercetin**: A flavonoid with strong antioxidant and anti-inflammatory effects[1].
- **Saponins**: These compounds have been shown to possess anti-inflammatory and immune-modulating properties[1].
- **Kaempferol**: Another flavonoid with antioxidant and anti-inflammatory activities[1].

Mechanisms of Action

- **Antioxidant Properties**: The compounds in hydrangea, such as hydrangin, quercetin, and kaempferol, help in scavenging free radicals and reducing oxidative stress. This is crucial in managing diabetes, as oxidative stress can damage pancreatic beta cells and impair insulin secretion[1].
- **Anti-inflammatory Effects**: Hydrangea's saponins and flavonoids reduce inflammation by inhibiting the production of pro-inflammatory cytokines. Chronic inflammation is a known contributor to insulin resistance and the progression of diabetes[1].
- **Improvement of Glucose Metabolism**: Some studies suggest that the compounds in hydrangea may help improve glucose metabolism by enhancing insulin sensitivity and reducing blood glucose levels[2].

Effects on Diabetes

- **Reduction of Blood Glucose Levels**: Hydrangea has been shown to significantly lower fasting blood glucose levels and improve glycemic control. This is achieved through its antioxidant and anti-inflammatory properties[2].

- **Improved Insulin Sensitivity**: By reducing oxidative stress and inflammation, hydrangea helps improve insulin sensitivity, which is crucial for effective glucose metabolism[2].
- **Cardiovascular Benefits**: The improvement in lipid profiles and reduction in oxidative stress contribute to better cardiovascular health, reducing the risk of complications associated with diabetes[2].

Dosages

The optimal dosage of hydrangea for managing diabetes is not well-established due to limited clinical studies. However, traditional usage and preliminary research suggest that doses ranging from **200 to 500 mg per day** of hydrangea root extract may be beneficial[3]. It is advisable to start with a lower dose and gradually increase it to monitor tolerance and effectiveness. Consulting with a healthcare provider before starting supplementation is recommended to tailor the dosage to individual needs and conditions[3].

Conclusion

Hydrangea, through its antioxidant, anti-inflammatory, and glucose metabolism-enhancing properties, offers potential therapeutic benefits for diabetes. Its mechanisms of action contribute to improved glycemic control, better lipid profiles, and protection against diabetic complications. While more research is needed to establish optimal dosages and long-term safety, current evidence supports the potential of hydrangea as a valuable supplement in managing diabetes.

Jujube

Jujube, also known as Chinese red dates, is a fruit with a long history of use in traditional Chinese medicine (TCM). It is known for its numerous health benefits, including its potential to regulate blood sugar levels and support overall health. Jujube has been used in TCM for over 2000 years. According to ancient Chinese texts, such as the "Treatise on Typhoid and Miscellaneous Diseases," jujube was used to strengthen the spleen and stomach, nourish the blood, and harmonize the body and mind[1]. It has also been used to treat various ailments, including anemia, insomnia, and digestive issues.

Active Ingredients and Compounds

Jujube contains several bioactive compounds, including polysaccharides, phenols, triterpene acids, flavonoids, polyphenols, vitamin C, tannins, and saponins[2]. These compounds contribute to jujube's antioxidant, anti-inflammatory, antimicrobial, and hypoglycemic properties.

Mechanism of Action

The primary mechanism by which jujube helps regulate blood sugar levels is through its low glycemic index (GI) and high dietary fiber content. Foods with a low GI are digested and absorbed more slowly, leading to a gradual rise in blood glucose levels[4]. The fiber in jujube slows the digestion and absorption of carbohydrates, preventing rapid increases in blood sugar levels. Additionally, jujube's bioactive compounds, such as polysaccharides and flavonoids, have been shown to improve insulin sensitivity and enhance glucose uptake in cells[3].

Doses

The recommended dose of jujube varies depending on the form and purpose of use. For fresh jujube, consuming 1-2 pieces per day is generally considered safe and beneficial. For dried jujube, a common dose is 10-15 grams per day, which can be consumed as a snack or brewed into tea[1]. It is important to consult with a healthcare provider before starting any new supplement regimen, especially for individuals with diabetes or other medical conditions.

Types and How to Supplement

Jujube is available in various forms, including fresh, dried, and as a supplement (capsules, powders, and extracts). Fresh jujube can be eaten as a snack or added to salads and desserts. Dried jujube can be used in cooking, baking, or brewed into tea. Supplements are convenient for those who prefer a more concentrated form and can be taken according to the manufacturer's instructions.

Conclusion

Jujube is a versatile fruit with numerous health benefits, particularly for individuals with diabetes. Its low GI, high fiber content, and bioactive compounds make it a valuable addition to a diabetic-friendly diet. By understanding its active ingredients, mechanism of action, history of use, and proper supplementation, individuals can harness the full potential of jujube to support their health.

Korean Ginseng

Korean ginseng, also known as Panax ginseng, has been used in traditional medicine for thousands of years, particularly in Asian cultures. It is renowned for its potential health benefits, including its role in managing diabetes and blood sugar levels.

Mechanisms of Action

- **Improving Insulin Sensitivity**: Korean ginseng has been shown to enhance insulin sensitivity, which is crucial for managing type 2 diabetes. It contains active compounds called ginsenosides that help improve the body's response to insulin[1]. By enhancing insulin sensitivity, Korean ginseng facilitates better glucose uptake by cells, thereby lowering blood sugar levels.
- **Regulating Blood Sugar Levels**: Studies have demonstrated that Korean ginseng can help regulate blood sugar levels by reducing fasting blood glucose and postprandial (after meal) blood glucose levels[2]. This is achieved through its ability to slow down carbohydrate absorption in the intestines and improve glucose metabolism.
- **Antioxidant and Anti-inflammatory Properties**: Chronic inflammation and oxidative stress are significant contributors to the development and progression of diabetes and its complications. Korean ginseng exhibits strong antioxidant and anti-inflammatory properties, which help reduce oxidative stress and inflammation[3]. This can protect pancreatic beta cells, which produce insulin, and improve overall metabolic health.

Clinical Evidence

Several studies have investigated the effects of Korean ginseng on diabetes management. For instance, a study published in the Journal of Ginseng Research found that Korean red ginseng significantly reduced fasting blood sugar levels and improved insulin sensitivity in people with type 2 diabetes[4]. Another study highlighted that Korean ginseng improved postprandial blood glucose levels and lipid profiles, suggesting its potential benefits for cardiovascular health as well.

Dosage and Safety

The typical dosage of Korean ginseng used in studies ranges from 200 to 400 mg per day, usually in the form of standardized extracts. It is generally well-tolerated, but some individuals may experience mild side effects such as headaches, digestive issues, or insomnia. It is important to consult with a healthcare provider before starting Korean ginseng supplementation, especially for individuals taking other medications, as ginseng can interact with certain drugs.

Conclusion

Korean ginseng offers several potential benefits for managing diabetes, particularly in improving insulin sensitivity, regulating blood sugar levels, and reducing oxidative stress and inflammation. While it is not a replacement for conventional diabetes treatments, Korean ginseng can be a valuable addition to a comprehensive diabetes management plan. As always, it is essential to discuss any new supplements with a healthcare provider to ensure they are safe and appropriate for individual health needs.

Lemon Balm

Lemon balm (Melissa officinalis) is a perennial herb belonging to the mint family, known for its calming and medicinal properties. Lemon balm has a long history of use in traditional medicine, dating back to ancient Greece and Rome. It was prescribed by doctors in the Middle Ages to improve sleep, reduce anxiety, and treat wounds[3]. The herb was also mentioned in classic literature, such as Homer's "The Odyssey" and by Persian writer Avicenna. In the 14th century, lemon balm was included in Carmelite water, an alcoholic extract beverage still sold in Germany today[3].

Effects on Blood Sugar and Diabetes

Lemon balm has shown potential in managing blood sugar levels and improving diabetes symptoms. Studies on animal models have demonstrated that lemon balm essential oil can significantly reduce blood glucose levels and improve glucose tolerance[2]. The essential oil increases the expression of glucose metabolism-related genes such as glucokinase and GLUT4, enhancing glucose uptake and metabolism in the liver and adipose tissue. Additionally, lemon balm has been found to increase insulin sensitivity and reduce oxidative stress related to diabetes[2].

Effects on Blood Pressure

Research on the effects of lemon balm on blood pressure is limited, but some studies suggest that it may help lower blood pressure. Animal studies have shown that lemon balm extract can reduce heart rate and blood pressure, potentially protecting the heart from injuries[3]. However, more research is needed to confirm these effects in humans.

Compounds and Mechanism of Action

Lemon balm contains several active compounds, including rosmarinic acid, ursolic acid, oleanolic acid, and various volatile compounds like geranial, neral, citronellal, and geraniol. These compounds have antioxidant, antimicrobial, and anti-inflammatory properties[5]. The primary mechanism of action involves increasing GABA (gamma-aminobutyric acid) levels in the brain, which produces a calming effect and reduces stress. Lemon balm also binds to nicotinic and muscarinic receptors in the brain, enhancing memory and alertness[4].

Recommended Doses

There is no official recommended daily allowance (RDA) for lemon balm, but clinical trials have studied doses ranging from 300 to 1,600 milligrams of lemon balm extract. It is important to consult a healthcare provider before using lemon balm supplements, especially if you are taking other medications or have underlying health conditions[5].

Conclusion

Lemon balm shows promise in managing blood sugar levels and improving diabetes symptoms, with potential benefits for blood pressure as well[3]. Its active compounds and mechanisms of action contribute to its calming and medicinal properties. With a rich history of use and ongoing research, lemon balm continues to be a valuable herb in natural medicine.

Leucine

Leucine is one of the nine essential amino acids required for protein synthesis and various metabolic functions in the human body. As a branched-chain amino acid (BCAA), leucine plays a crucial role not only in muscle protein synthesis but also in regulating glucose metabolism. Emerging research has highlighted leucine's potential therapeutic effects on diabetes, particularly Type 2 diabetes mellitus (T2DM).

History of Leucine

Leucine was first isolated in 1819 by the French chemist Joseph Louis Proust from cheese. Later, in 1820, Henri Braconnot extracted it from muscle fiber and wool. Its importance was not fully understood until the 20th century when its role as an essential amino acid was established. As research advanced, leucine was identified as a critical regulator of muscle protein synthesis and metabolic pathways influencing glucose homeostasis.

Leucine affects glucose metabolism through several mechanisms:

- **Stimulation of Insulin Secretion**

- **Pancreatic β-Cells Activation**: Leucine stimulates insulin secretion from pancreatic β-cells. It does so by enhancing the mitochondrial production of ATP, which in turn closes ATP-sensitive potassium channels, leading to cell membrane depolarization and insulin release.

- **Activation of the mTOR Pathway**

- **mTOR Signaling**: Leucine activates the mammalian target of rapamycin (mTOR) pathway, which is crucial for protein synthesis and cell growth. Activation of mTOR improves insulin signaling and promotes glucose uptake in muscle cells.

- **Gluconeogenesis Regulation**

- **Inhibition of Gluconeogenesis**: Leucine suppresses gluconeogenesis in the liver by influencing key enzymes, thereby reducing hepatic glucose production.

- **Enhancement of Glucose Uptake**

- **Glucose Transporters**: Leucine increases the translocation of glucose transporter type 4 (GLUT4) to the cell membrane in muscle tissue, enhancing glucose uptake independent of insulin action.

How Leucine Helps in Diabetes Management

- **Improving Glycemic Control**

- **Enhanced Insulin Secretion**: By stimulating insulin release, leucine helps lower blood glucose levels.

- **Increased Glucose Uptake**: Leucine-mediated GLUT4 translocation facilitates glucose absorption by muscle cells.

- **Reducing Insulin Resistance**

- **mTOR Activation**: Improved insulin signaling through mTOR activation can reduce insulin resistance, a key feature of T2DM.

- **Preserving Muscle Mass**

- **Protein Synthesis**: Leucine promotes muscle protein synthesis, which is beneficial as muscle mass is inversely related to insulin resistance.

- **Suppressing Appetite**

- **Satiety Signals**: Leucine influences the hypothalamus to promote satiety, which may help in weight management, an important aspect of T2DM control.

Types of Leucine Supplementation

- **Free-Form L-Leucine Supplements**

- **Description**: Pure leucine without any additional amino acids.

- **Usage**: Often used to stimulate muscle protein synthesis and support metabolic health.

- **Branched-Chain Amino Acid (BCAA) Supplements**

- **Composition**: Contains leucine, isoleucine, and valine in varying ratios.

- **Usage**: Popular among athletes to enhance performance and recovery; may also benefit glucose metabolism.

- **Whey Protein Supplements**

- **Content**: High in leucine along with other essential amino acids.

- **Usage**: Supports muscle growth and has been shown to improve postprandial glucose levels.

- **Leucine-Enriched Meal Replacements**

- **Description**: Nutritional shakes or bars fortified with additional leucine.

- **Usage**: Aimed at providing balanced nutrition with metabolic benefits.

Recommended Doses

- **General Guidance: Leucine** Alone: Daily supplementation of 2-5 grams of free-form leucine. **BCAA Supplements**: Typically, 5-10 grams per dose, containing leucine in combination with isoleucine and valine. **Whey Protein**: Serving sizes vary, but aim for a leucine content of 2-3 grams per serving.

- ## Considerations:

- **Timing**: Taking leucine with meals may enhance its insulinotropic effects. **Individual Needs**: Dosage may vary based on body weight, activity level, and metabolic health. Consulting a healthcare provider is recommended.

Safety and Potential Side Effects

- **General Safety**: Leucine is generally considered safe when consumed within recommended doses.

- **Excess Intake**: Very high doses may lead to adverse effects such as hypoglycemia, ammonia accumulation, or interfere with other amino acids' absorption.

- **Interactions**: Individuals with maple syrup urine disease or other metabolic disorders should avoid leucine supplementation unless under medical supervision.

Conclusion

Leucine, an essential branched-chain amino acid, has demonstrated significant potential in managing diabetes through various mechanisms. By stimulating insulin secretion, enhancing insulin signaling via the mTOR pathway, and promoting glucose uptake, leucine can improve glycemic control and reduce insulin resistance. Supplementation with leucine, whether as free-form, part of BCAA supplements, or through leucine-rich foods like whey protein, may offer therapeutic benefits for individuals with Type 2 diabetes. However, it is important to consider appropriate dosing and consult healthcare professionals to tailor supplementation to individual needs.

Licorice Root

Licorice root, derived from the root of the Glycyrrhiza glabra plant, has been used medicinally for thousands of years.

Active Ingredients and Compounds

Licorice root contains over 300 chemical compounds, with the primary active compound being **glycyrrhizin**. Other significant compounds include **triterpenoid saponins**, **flavonoids**, and **polysaccharides**. These compounds are known for their antioxidant, anti-inflammatory, and antimicrobial properties[3].

Mechanism of Action

The active compounds in licorice root, particularly glycyrrhizin, exert their effects through several mechanisms. Glycyrrhizin has been shown to **reduce blood glucose levels** by inhibiting the enzyme **11-beta-hydroxysteroid dehydrogenase**[1], which leads to increased insulin sensitivity and improved glucose uptake by cells. Additionally, licorice root has been found to **reduce inflammation** and **protect pancreatic beta cells**, which are crucial for insulin production.

History of Use

Licorice root has a long history of medicinal use dating back to ancient Egypt, where it was made into a sweet drink for pharaohs. It has been used in traditional Chinese medicine for treating various ailments, including **gastrointestinal problems, respiratory infections, and inflammation**[1]. Licorice root was also widely used in Europe and Asia for its therapeutic properties.

Doses

The recommended dose of licorice root varies depending on the form and purpose of use. For general health benefits, a typical dose is **250-500 mg of licorice root extract** taken **1-2 times daily**. However, it is essential to consult a healthcare provider before starting any supplementation, especially for individuals with pre-existing health conditions.

Types and How to Supplement

Licorice root is available in various forms, including capsules, teas, tinctures, and extracts. When choosing a supplement, it is crucial to select a product that is standardized for glycyrrhizin content to ensure consistency and efficacy[3]. Licorice root supplements should be taken with caution, as **excessive consumption can lead to adverse effects such as high blood pressure and water retention**.

Conclusion

Licorice root has shown promising potential in managing diabetes and regulating blood sugar levels due to its active compounds and mechanisms of action. However, it is essential to use it under the guidance of a healthcare provider to avoid potential side effects and ensure safe and effective use.

Magnesium

Magnesium is an essential mineral involved in numerous bodily functions, including muscle and nerve function, blood glucose control, and bone health. It plays a particularly important role in managing diabetes, especially type 2 diabetes. Research has shown that adequate magnesium intake is crucial for maintaining metabolic health and preventing diabetes-related complications. It is important to buy a better-quality magnesium supplement, such as Magnesium Taurate, citrate, Threonate, orotate, aspartate, glycinate.

Mechanisms of Action

- **Improving Insulin Sensitivity**: Magnesium is vital for insulin signaling and glucose uptake. It acts as a cofactor for various enzymes involved in carbohydrate metabolism. Adequate magnesium levels help improve insulin sensitivity, allowing cells to use glucose more effectively and lowering blood sugar levels[1]. This is particularly beneficial for people with insulin resistance, a common feature of type 2 diabetes.
- **Regulating Blood Sugar Levels**: Magnesium helps regulate blood sugar levels by influencing the activity of insulin receptors and enhancing the action of insulin[2]. It also plays a role in the secretion of insulin from the pancreas, ensuring that the body can respond appropriately to rising blood glucose levels after meals[3].
- **Reducing Inflammation and Oxidative Stress**: Chronic inflammation and oxidative stress are significant contributors to the development and progression of diabetes and its complications. Magnesium has anti-inflammatory and antioxidant properties that help reduce inflammation and protect cells from oxidative damage[4]. This can help prevent complications such as cardiovascular disease and neuropathy.

Clinical Evidence

Several studies have highlighted the benefits of magnesium for diabetes management. **For instance, a meta-analysis of 13 prospective cohort studies involving over 500,000 participants found that higher magnesium intake was associated with a lower risk of developing type 2 diabetes[5].** Another study published in Diabetes Care found that magnesium supplementation improved insulin sensitivity and glycemic control in people with type 2 diabetes[6].

Dosage and Safety

The recommended daily allowance (RDA) for magnesium varies by age and sex, but for adults, it generally ranges from 310 to 420 mg per day. Magnesium can be obtained from dietary sources such as leafy green vegetables, nuts, seeds, whole grains, and legumes. For those who have difficulty meeting their magnesium needs through diet alone, supplements are available. It is important to consult with a healthcare provider before starting magnesium supplementation, especially for individuals with kidney disease or those taking other medications, as high doses of magnesium can cause adverse effects[7].

Conclusion

Magnesium plays a crucial role in managing diabetes by improving insulin sensitivity, regulating blood sugar levels, and reducing inflammation and oxidative stress. While it is not a replacement for conventional diabetes treatments, adequate magnesium intake can be a valuable component of a comprehensive diabetes management plan. As always, it is essential to discuss any new supplements with a healthcare provider to ensure they are safe and appropriate for individual health needs.

Milk Thistle

Milk thistle (Silybum marianum) is a flowering herb known for its medicinal properties, particularly for liver health. Recent studies have suggested that milk thistle may also have beneficial effects on diabetes and blood sugar control.

Active Ingredients and Compounds

The primary active ingredient in milk thistle is **silymarin,** a complex of flavonoids, including **silibinin, silydianin, and silychristin**. These compounds are known for their antioxidant, anti-inflammatory, and hepatoprotective properties.

Mechanism of Action

Milk thistle's hypoglycemic effects are attributed to its ability to improve insulin sensitivity and reduce oxidative stress. Silymarin helps to **protect pancreatic beta cells**, which are responsible for insulin production[2]. By reducing inflammation and oxidative stress, milk thistle supports overall metabolic health and helps regulate blood sugar levels.

History of Use

Milk thistle has been used for over 2,000 years in traditional medicine for its liver-protective properties. It was first documented in ancient Greek and Roman texts and has been a staple in herbal medicine ever since[1]. In modern times, milk thistle is widely used to support liver health and is being studied for its potential benefits in managing diabetes.

Doses

The recommended dose of milk thistle varies depending on the form and purpose of use. For diabetes management, studies have shown that **140 mg of silymarin extract** taken **three times daily** can be effective. It's important to consult with a healthcare provider before starting any new supplement regimen to ensure safety and effectiveness.

Types and How to Supplement

Milk thistle is available in various forms, including capsules, tablets, liquid extracts, and teas. To supplement with milk thistle, you can:

- Take capsules or tablets as directed by a healthcare provider.
- Brew milk thistle tea by steeping the dried herb in hot water.
- Use liquid extracts according to the manufacturer's instructions.

Conclusion

Milk thistle shows promise as a natural supplement for managing diabetes and regulating blood sugar levels. Its active compounds, particularly silymarin, contribute to its hypoglycemic and antioxidant properties[1]. With a long history of use in traditional medicine and various forms available for supplementation, milk thistle is a versatile and accessible option for those looking to improve their health.

Nattokinase

Nattokinase is an enzyme extracted from natto, a traditional Japanese food made from fermented soybeans. Known for its fibrinolytic (clot-dissolving) properties, nattokinase has been studied for various health benefits, including its potential effects on blood sugar control and diabetes management.

Mechanisms of Action

- **Improving Insulin Sensitivity**: Nattokinase has been shown to enhance insulin sensitivity, which is crucial for managing type 2 diabetes. By improving the body's response to insulin, nattokinase helps cells absorb glucose more efficiently, thereby lowering blood sugar levels[1].
- **Regulating Blood Sugar Levels**: Nattokinase may help regulate blood sugar levels by influencing metabolic pathways involved in glucose metabolism. It has been observed to lower fasting blood glucose levels and improve overall glucose tolerance[2]. This regulation helps maintain stable blood sugar levels and prevents hyperglycemia.
- **Anti-inflammatory Properties**: Chronic inflammation is a significant contributor to the development and progression of diabetes. Nattokinase exhibits anti-inflammatory properties that help reduce inflammation in the body[3]. By mitigating inflammation, nattokinase can improve insulin sensitivity and overall metabolic health.

Clinical Evidence

Several studies have investigated the effects of nattokinase on diabetes management. **For instance, a study published in the Journal of Endocrine Society found that nattokinase supplementation improved HbA1c, fasting insulin, glucose levels, and HOMA-IR scores in individuals with metabolic syndrome[4]**. These findings suggest that nattokinase can be beneficial for improving blood sugar control and insulin sensitivity.
Another study highlighted that nattokinase's probiotic properties might boost metabolism and reduce body fat, potentially preventing metabolic disorders like obesity and diabetes[2]. This indicates that nattokinase could play a role in both the prevention and management of diabetes.

Dosage and Safety

The typical dosage of nattokinase used in studies ranges from 100 to 200 mg per day. It is generally well-tolerated, but some individuals may experience mild side effects such as gastrointestinal discomfort or allergic reactions[5]. It is important to consult with a healthcare provider before starting nattokinase supplementation, especially for individuals taking other medications, as nattokinase can interact with certain drugs and increase the risk of bleeding.

Conclusion

Nattokinase offers several potential benefits for managing diabetes, particularly in improving insulin sensitivity, regulating blood sugar levels, and reducing inflammation. While it is not a replacement for conventional diabetes treatments, nattokinase can be a valuable addition to a comprehensive diabetes management plan. As always, it is essential to discuss any new supplements with a healthcare provider to ensure they are safe and appropriate for individual health needs.

Nitrosigine

Nitrosigine, a patented complex of arginine and silicon, is known for its potential benefits in enhancing nitric oxide levels, improving blood flow, and supporting cardiovascular health. Recent studies have explored its potential effects on diabetes and neuropathy.

Compounds Derived from Nitrosigine

- **Arginine**: An amino acid that plays a crucial role in the production of nitric oxide, which helps in vasodilation and improving blood flow[1].
- **Silicon**: A trace element that supports the structural integrity of blood vessels and enhances the bioavailability of arginine[1].

Mechanisms of Action

- **Nitric Oxide Production**: Arginine in nitrosigine is a precursor to nitric oxide (NO), a molecule that promotes vasodilation and improves blood flow. Enhanced NO production can help improve circulation, which is beneficial for managing diabetes and its complications[1].
- **Improved Blood Flow**: By increasing NO levels, nitrosigine helps improve blood flow to peripheral tissues, which can alleviate symptoms of diabetic neuropathy by ensuring better oxygen and nutrient delivery to damaged nerves[1].
- **Anti-inflammatory Effects**: Nitrosigine has been shown to reduce inflammation by modulating the activity of pro-inflammatory cytokines. Chronic inflammation is a known contributor to insulin resistance and the progression of diabetes[2].
- **Antioxidant Properties**: Nitrosigine helps reduce oxidative stress by enhancing the body's antioxidant defenses. This is crucial in managing diabetes, as oxidative stress can damage pancreatic beta cells and impair insulin secretion[2].

Effects on Diabetes

- **Improved Glycemic Control**: By enhancing blood flow and reducing inflammation, nitrosigine can help improve insulin sensitivity and glucose metabolism, leading to better glycemic control[2].

- **Cardiovascular Benefits**: Improved nitric oxide production and reduced oxidative stress contribute to better cardiovascular health, reducing the risk of complications associated with diabetes[2].
- **Protection Against Diabetic Complications**: The antioxidant and anti-inflammatory properties of nitrosigine help protect against complications such as diabetic neuropathy, nephropathy, and retinopathy[2].

Effects on Neuropathy

- **Pain Reduction**: Improved blood flow and reduced inflammation can help alleviate neuropathic pain by ensuring better oxygen and nutrient delivery to damaged nerves[2].
- **Nerve Regeneration**: Enhanced circulation and reduced oxidative stress support nerve repair and regeneration, which is crucial for managing neuropathy[2].
- **Improved Sensory Function**: By reducing inflammation and oxidative damage, nitrosigine helps improve sensory and motor functions in individuals with neuropathy[2].

Dosages

The optimal dosage of nitrosigine for managing diabetes and neuropathy varies, but studies suggest that doses ranging from **750 to 1500 mg per day** are generally safe and effective[2]. It is advisable to start with a lower dose and gradually increase it to monitor tolerance and effectiveness. Consulting with a healthcare provider before starting supplementation is recommended to tailor the dosage to individual needs and conditions[2].

Conclusion

Nitrosigine, through its nitric oxide-enhancing, anti-inflammatory, and antioxidant properties, offers significant therapeutic benefits for diabetes and neuropathy. Its mechanisms of action contribute to improved glycemic control, better cardiovascular health, and protection against diabetic complications. While more research is needed to establish optimal dosages and long-term safety, current evidence supports the potential of nitrosigine as a valuable supplement in managing diabetes and neuropathy.

NO3-T Creatine Nitrate

NO3-T creatine nitrate is a patented blend of creatine and nitrate, designed to enhance the benefits of both compounds. This is usually found in preworkout powders as it's a NO booster.

Compounds Derived from NO3-T Creatine Nitrate

- **Creatine**: An amino acid derivative that plays a crucial role in energy production, particularly in muscle cells[1].
- **Nitrate**: A compound that can be converted into nitric oxide (NO) in the body, which helps in vasodilation and improving blood flow[1].

Mechanisms of Action

- **Nitric Oxide Production**: The nitrate component of NO3-T creatine nitrate is converted into nitric oxide (NO) in the body. NO is a potent vasodilator, which means it helps relax blood vessels and improve blood flow. Enhanced NO production can improve circulation, which is beneficial for managing diabetes and its complications[1].
- **Improved Blood Flow**: By increasing NO levels, NO3-T creatine nitrate helps improve blood flow to peripheral tissues. This can alleviate symptoms of diabetic neuropathy by ensuring better oxygen and nutrient delivery to damaged nerves[1].
- **Enhanced Glucose Uptake**: Creatine has been shown to enhance glucose uptake in muscle cells by increasing the translocation of glucose transporter type 4 (GLUT4) to the cell membrane. This can help lower blood glucose levels and improve insulin sensitivity[2].
- **Anti-inflammatory Effects**: NO3-T creatine nitrate has been shown to reduce inflammation by modulating the activity of pro-inflammatory cytokines. Chronic inflammation is a known contributor to insulin resistance and the progression of diabetes[2].
- **Antioxidant Properties**: The combination of creatine and nitrate helps reduce oxidative stress by enhancing the body's antioxidant defenses. This is crucial in managing diabetes, as oxidative stress can damage pancreatic beta cells and impair insulin secretion[2].

Effects on Diabetes

- **Improved Glycemic Control**: By enhancing blood flow, reducing inflammation, and improving glucose uptake, NO3-T creatine nitrate can help improve insulin sensitivity and glucose metabolism, leading to better glycemic control[2].
- **Cardiovascular Benefits**: Improved nitric oxide production and reduced oxidative stress contribute to better cardiovascular health, reducing the risk of complications associated with diabetes[2].
- **Protection Against Diabetic Complications**: The antioxidant and anti-inflammatory properties of NO3-T creatine nitrate help protect against complications such as diabetic neuropathy, nephropathy, and retinopathy[2].

Dosages

The optimal dosage of NO3-T creatine nitrate for managing diabetes varies, but studies suggest that doses ranging from **750 to 1500 mg per day** are generally safe and effective[2]. It is advisable to start with a lower dose and gradually increase it to monitor tolerance and effectiveness. Consulting with a healthcare provider before starting supplementation is recommended to tailor the dosage to individual needs and conditions[2].

Conclusion

NO3-T creatine nitrate, through its nitric oxide-enhancing, anti-inflammatory, and antioxidant properties, offers significant therapeutic benefits for diabetes. Its mechanisms of action contribute to improved glycemic control, better cardiovascular health, and protection against diabetic complications. While more research is needed to establish optimal dosages and long-term safety, current evidence supports the potential of NO3-T creatine nitrate as a valuable supplement in managing diabetes.

Plantain (Plantago major)

Plantain (Plantago major) is a perennial herb widely recognized for its medicinal properties. Traditionally used in various cultures for its healing benefits, recent studies have explored its potential in managing diabetes.

Plantago major has been used in traditional medicine across different cultures. Native Americans utilized it for wound healing, respiratory issues, and digestive problems. In European folk medicine, it was commonly used for its anti-inflammatory and antimicrobial properties[1]. The leaves, seeds, and roots of the plant were often prepared as teas, poultices, or extracts to treat various ailments.

Compounds Derived from Plantago major

- **Iridoid Glycosides**: These compounds, including aucubin and catalpol, are known for their anti-inflammatory and antimicrobial properties[2].
- **Flavonoids**: Plantago major contains flavonoids such as **apigenin** and **luteolin**, which have antioxidant and anti-inflammatory effects[3].
- **Polysaccharides**: These compounds contribute to the plant's immunomodulatory and wound-healing properties[4].
- **Phenolic Acids**: Compounds like caffeic acid and chlorogenic acid exhibit strong antioxidant activities[5].

Mechanisms of Action

- **Antioxidant Properties**: The phenolic acids and flavonoids in Plantago major help in scavenging free radicals and reducing oxidative stress, which is crucial in managing diabetes as oxidative stress can damage pancreatic beta cells and impair insulin secretion[5].
- **Anti-inflammatory Effects**: Iridoid glycosides and flavonoids reduce inflammation by inhibiting the production of pro-inflammatory cytokines. Chronic inflammation is a known contributor to insulin resistance and the progression of diabetes[2].
- **Inhibition of Carbohydrate-Digesting Enzymes**: Plantago major has been shown to inhibit the activity of α-amylase and α-glucosidase, enzymes involved in the breakdown of carbohydrates. This inhibition slows down the absorption of glucose, leading to lower postprandial blood glucose levels[3].

- **Improvement of Lipid Profiles**: The plant's compounds help in reducing total cholesterol, LDL cholesterol, and triglycerides, which are often elevated in diabetic patients[4].

Effects on Diabetes

- **Reduction of Blood Glucose Levels**: Plantago major has been shown to significantly lower fasting and postprandial blood glucose levels. This is achieved through its antioxidant, anti-inflammatory, and enzyme-inhibiting properties[3].
- **Improved Insulin Sensitivity**: By reducing oxidative stress and inflammation, Plantago major helps improve insulin sensitivity, which is crucial for effective glucose metabolism[2].
- **Cardiovascular Benefits**: The improvement in lipid profiles and reduction in oxidative stress contribute to better cardiovascular health, reducing the risk of complications associated with diabetes[4].
- **Protection Against Diabetic Complications**: The antioxidant and anti-inflammatory properties of Plantago major help protect against complications such as diabetic neuropathy, nephropathy, and retinopathy[5].

Dosages

The optimal dosage of Plantago major for managing diabetes varies, but studies suggest that doses ranging from **300 to 600 mg per day** are generally safe and effective[4]. It is advisable to start with a lower dose and gradually increase it to monitor tolerance and effectiveness. Consulting with a healthcare provider before starting supplementation is recommended to tailor the dosage to individual needs and conditions[4].

Conclusion

Plantago major, through its antioxidant, anti-inflammatory, and enzyme-inhibiting properties, offers significant therapeutic benefits for diabetes. Its mechanisms of action contribute to improved glycemic control, better lipid profiles, and protection against diabetic complications. While more research is needed to establish optimal dosages and long-term safety, current evidence supports the potential of Plantago major as a valuable supplement in managing diabetes.

Poria

Poria (**Poria cocos**), also known as **Fu Ling** in Traditional Chinese Medicine (TCM), is a fungus that grows on the roots of pine trees. It has been used for centuries in TCM for its diuretic, sedative, and tonic properties. Recently, interest has grown in its potential effects on diabetes and blood sugar regulation.

Active Ingredients and Compounds

Poria contains several bioactive compounds that contribute to its medicinal properties:

- **Polysaccharides**: The most abundant constituents, including Pachyman, which have immunomodulatory and hypoglycemic effects.
- **Triterpenoids**: Such as pachymic acid and poricoic acids, known for anti-inflammatory and antioxidant activities.
- **Ergosterol**: A sterol that can be converted into vitamin D_2 and has antioxidant properties.
- **Adenine and Choline**: Compounds that may support metabolic processes.

Mechanism of Action

The potential hypoglycemic effects of Poria are attributed to its polysaccharides and triterpenoids:

- **Enhancing Insulin Sensitivity**: Poria polysaccharides may improve insulin receptor function, enhancing glucose uptake by cells.
- **Regulating Glucose Metabolism**: By influencing enzymes involved in glucose metabolism, Poria may help stabilize blood sugar levels.
- **Anti-Inflammatory Effects**: Triterpenoids reduce inflammation, which is often associated with insulin resistance.
- **Antioxidant Activity**: The compounds scavenge free radicals, protecting pancreatic beta cells from oxidative damage.

History of Use

- **Traditional Chinese Medicine**: Poria has been used for over 2,000 years in TCM. It appears in classic texts like the "Shennong Ben Cao Jing" as a top-grade herb.
- **Applications in TCM**: Traditionally used to promote urination, strengthen the spleen, harmonize the middle burner (digestive system), and calm the mind.
- **Formulas**: Commonly included in herbal formulas for edema, diarrhea, palpitations, insomnia, and spleen deficiency.

Doses

- **Decoction**: Typical doses range from **9 to 15 grams** of dried Poria, boiled in water.
- **Powdered Extracts**: **1 to 3 grams** per day, standardized extracts providing specific amounts of polysaccharides.
- **Capsules/Tablets**: Follow manufacturer's recommendations, usually **500 mg** taken **2-3 times daily**.

Types and How to Supplement

- **Whole Dried Sclerotium**: Used in decoctions; boiled to extract active compounds.
- **Powdered Extracts**: Standardized for polysaccharide content; offers convenience and consistent dosing.
- **Capsules/Tablets**: Easy ingestion; may combine Poria with other complementary herbs.
- **Teas**: Poria can be steeped to make herbal teas, often blended with other herbs.

Supplementation Tips:

- **Quality Assurance**: Choose supplements from reputable companies that perform quality testing for purity and potency.
- **Standardization**: Look for products standardized to contain a specific percentage of polysaccharides.
- **Professional Guidance**: Consult with a healthcare provider or a practitioner of TCM for personalized advice, especially if taking other medications.

Conclusion

Poria (**Poria cocos**) holds potential benefits for supporting blood sugar regulation and managing diabetes, primarily due to its polysaccharides and triterpenoids. Its long history in Traditional Chinese Medicine underscores its importance as a medicinal fungus. While preliminary studies are promising, further clinical research is needed to fully establish its efficacy and optimal usage guidelines. Individuals interested in using Poria should seek professional advice to ensure safe and effective supplementation.

Psyllium Husk

Psyllium husk, derived from the seeds of the Plantago ovata plant, is a type of soluble fiber that has gained popularity for its numerous health benefits, particularly in managing blood sugar levels.

Mechanisms of Action

- **Slowing Glucose Absorption**: Psyllium husk forms a viscous gel when mixed with water, which slows the digestion and absorption of carbohydrates in the small intestine[1]. This delayed absorption helps prevent rapid spikes in blood sugar levels after meals, leading to more stable blood glucose levels.
- **Delaying Gastric Emptying**: The gel-like substance formed by psyllium husk also slows down the rate at which food leaves the stomach[2]. This extended digestion time allows for a more gradual release of glucose into the bloodstream, helping to maintain steady blood sugar levels.
- **Enhancing Insulin Sensitivity**: Regular consumption of psyllium husk has been shown to improve insulin sensitivity[3]. By enhancing the body's response to insulin, psyllium helps cells absorb glucose more efficiently, reducing overall blood sugar levels.

Clinical Evidence

Several studies have demonstrated the efficacy of psyllium husk in managing blood sugar levels. For instance, a study published in Diabetes Care found that taking 5.1 grams of psyllium husk twice daily for eight weeks significantly reduced fasting blood glucose levels and HbA1c, a marker of long-term blood sugar control[1]. Participants experienced an average reduction of 52.6 mg/dL in fasting glucose levels and a 1.6% decrease in HbA1c levels.
Another study highlighted that psyllium husk supplementation improved postprandial (after meal) blood glucose levels in people with type 2 diabetes[2]. The study found that psyllium husk reduced the glycemic response to meals, leading to lower blood sugar spikes.

Dosage and Safety

The typical dosage of psyllium husk used in studies ranges from 5 to 15 grams per day, usually taken before meals. It is generally well-tolerated, but some individuals may experience mild gastrointestinal side effects such as bloating or gas[3]. It is important to start with a lower dose and gradually increase it to allow the body to adjust. Additionally, it is essential to drink plenty of water when taking psyllium husk to prevent digestive discomfort.

Conclusion

Psyllium husk offers several potential benefits for managing blood sugar levels, particularly in slowing glucose absorption, delaying gastric emptying, and enhancing insulin sensitivity. While it is not a replacement for conventional diabetes treatments, psyllium husk can be a valuable addition to a comprehensive diabetes management plan. As always, it is essential to discuss any new supplements with a healthcare provider to ensure they are safe and appropriate for individual health needs.

Raspberry Extract

Raspberry extract, derived from the fruit of the raspberry plant, is rich in antioxidants, vitamins, and fiber. It has gained attention for its potential health benefits, particularly in managing blood sugar levels and diabetes.

Mechanisms of Action

- **Improving Insulin Sensitivity**: Raspberry extract contains bioactive compounds such as anthocyanins and ellagitannins, which have been shown to enhance insulin sensitivity[1]. By improving the body's response to insulin, these compounds help cells absorb glucose more efficiently, thereby lowering blood sugar levels.
- **Regulating Blood Sugar Levels**: The fiber content in raspberry extract helps slow the digestion and absorption of carbohydrates[2]. This delayed absorption prevents rapid spikes in blood sugar levels after meals, leading to more stable blood glucose levels throughout the day.
- **Anti-inflammatory and Antioxidant Properties**: Chronic inflammation and oxidative stress are significant contributors to the development and progression of diabetes. Raspberry extract exhibits strong anti-inflammatory and antioxidant properties, which help reduce inflammation and protect cells from oxidative damage[3]. This can improve overall metabolic health and prevent complications associated with diabetes.

Clinical Evidence

Several studies have demonstrated the efficacy of raspberry extract in managing blood sugar levels. For instance, a study conducted by the Illinois Institute of Technology found that consuming red raspberries reduced the amount of insulin needed to manage blood glucose levels in individuals with pre-diabetes[1]. The study showed that as the amount of raspberry intake increased, glucose concentrations were lower compared to meals without raspberries.

Another study published in the International Journal of Environmental Research and Public Health highlighted that red raspberries contain various phytonutrients that can modulate insulin function, glucose, and lipid metabolism[4]. The review suggested that red raspberries might offer clinically beneficial effects for the prevention and management of chronic diseases through improvements in glucose handling and insulin sensitivity.

Dosage and Safety

The typical dosage of raspberry extract used in studies varies, but it is generally considered safe when consumed in amounts found in food. Some individuals may experience mild gastrointestinal discomfort if taken in large quantities[5]. It is important to consult with a healthcare provider before starting raspberry extract supplementation, especially for individuals taking other medications, as it can interact with certain drugs.

Conclusion

Raspberry extract offers several potential benefits for managing diabetes, particularly in improving insulin sensitivity, regulating blood sugar levels, and reducing inflammation and oxidative stress. While it is not a replacement for conventional diabetes treatments, raspberry extract can be a valuable addition to a comprehensive diabetes management plan. As always, it is essential to discuss any new supplements with a healthcare provider to ensure they are safe and appropriate for individual health needs.

Rehmannia

Rehmannia, also known as Chinese foxglove or Rehmannia glutinosa, is a perennial plant native to China. It has been used in Traditional Chinese Medicine (TCM) for centuries to treat various health conditions, including diabetes[1]. Rehmannia has a long history of use in TCM, dating back over 1,000 years. It is considered one of the top 50 fundamental herbs in TCM and is often used in combination with other herbs to treat various conditions, including diabetes[1]. In Japanese medicine, Rehmannia is also used as a general tonic to improve overall health.

Active Ingredients and Compounds

- **Tyrosol**: An antioxidant that helps reduce oxidative stress.
- **Acteoside**: A phenylethanoid glycoside with anti-inflammatory and antioxidant properties.
- **Leucosceptoside A**: A phenylethanoid glycoside that exhibits anti-inflammatory effects.
- **Martynoside**: A phenylethanoid glycoside with antioxidant properties.
- **Isomartynoside**: A phenylethanoid glycoside with anti-inflammatory effects.
- **Purpureaside C**: A phenylethanoid glycoside with antioxidant properties.
- **Jionoside A1 and B1**: Phenylethanoid glycosides with anti-inflammatory effects.

Mechanism of Action

- **Antioxidant Activity**: The phenylethanoid glycosides and other compounds in Rehmannia help reduce oxidative stress, which is a contributing factor in the development of diabetes.
- **Anti-inflammatory Effects**: The anti-inflammatory properties of Rehmannia help reduce inflammation in the body, which can improve insulin sensitivity and glucose metabolism.
- **Blood Sugar Regulation**: Rehmannia has been shown to lower blood sugar levels by enhancing insulin secretion and improving insulin sensitivity.

Doses

The appropriate dose of Rehmannia can vary depending on the individual's condition and the form of Rehmannia used. Common doses include:

- **Tea**: 1-2 teaspoons of dried Rehmannia root per cup of boiling water, steeped for 10-15 minutes.
- **Capsules**: 500-1,000 mg of Rehmannia extract per day, divided into 2-3 doses.
- **Tincture**: 2-4 ml of Rehmannia tincture (1:2 or 1:5) per day, diluted in water or juice.

Types and How to Supplement

- **Consult a Healthcare Professional**: Before starting any new supplement, it's important to consult with a healthcare professional to ensure it's safe and appropriate for your condition.
- **Choose the Right Form**: Select the form of Rehmannia that best suits your needs and preferences.
- **Follow Dosage Instructions**: Take the recommended dose as directed on the product label or by your healthcare professional.
- **Monitor Your Health**: Keep track of any changes in your blood sugar levels and overall health while taking Rehmannia.

Conclusion

Rehmannia is a valuable herb in TCM with potential benefits for managing diabetes and blood sugar levels. Its active compounds, antioxidant and anti-inflammatory properties, and history of use make it a promising natural remedy. However, it's important to consult with a healthcare professional before using Rehmannia as a supplement.

Resveratrol

Resveratrol is a naturally occurring polyphenolic compound found in various plants, including grapes, berries, and peanuts. It is most famously associated with red wine. Over the past few decades, resveratrol has garnered significant attention for its potential health benefits, particularly in managing diabetes and blood sugar levels.

Mechanisms of Action

- **Improving Insulin Sensitivity**: Resveratrol has been shown to enhance insulin sensitivity, which is crucial for managing type 2 diabetes. It activates AMP-activated protein kinase (AMPK), an enzyme that plays a key role in cellular energy homeostasis. By activating AMPK, resveratrol helps improve the body's response to insulin, facilitating better glucose uptake by cells and lowering blood sugar levels[1].
- **Regulating Glucose Metabolism**: Resveratrol influences several pathways involved in glucose metabolism. It promotes glycolysis, the process by which glucose is broken down to produce energy, and inhibits gluconeogenesis, the production of glucose in the liver[2]. These actions help maintain stable blood sugar levels and prevent hyperglycemia.
- **Antioxidant and Anti-inflammatory Properties**: Chronic inflammation and oxidative stress are significant contributors to the development and progression of diabetes and its complications. Resveratrol's potent antioxidant properties help neutralize free radicals, reducing oxidative stress and inflammation[3]. This can protect pancreatic beta cells, which produce insulin, and improve overall metabolic health.

Clinical Evidence

Several studies have investigated the effects of resveratrol on diabetes management. For instance, a comprehensive review published in Molecular Biology Reports highlighted that resveratrol limits glucose absorption in the intestines, promotes glycogen formation in the liver, boosts insulin secretion in pancreatic cells, enhances insulin receptiveness in muscle cells, and inhibits triglyceride production in fat cells[3]. These multifaceted effects contribute to better glucose homeostasis and metabolic health.
Another study published in Diabetes Care found that resveratrol supplementation improved glucose control and insulin sensitivity in people

with type 2 diabetes[4]. Participants who took resveratrol showed significant reductions in fasting blood glucose levels and HbA1c, a marker of long-term blood sugar control.

Dosage and Safety

The typical dosage of resveratrol used in studies ranges from 150 to 500 mg per day. It is generally well-tolerated, but some individuals may experience mild side effects such as gastrointestinal discomfort. It is important to consult with a healthcare provider before starting resveratrol supplementation, especially for those taking other medications, as resveratrol can interact with certain drugs[5].

Conclusion

Resveratrol offers several potential benefits for managing diabetes, particularly in improving insulin sensitivity, regulating glucose metabolism, and reducing oxidative stress and inflammation. While it is not a replacement for conventional diabetes treatments, resveratrol can be a valuable addition to a comprehensive diabetes management plan. As always, it is essential to discuss any new supplements with a healthcare provider to ensure they are safe and appropriate for individual health needs.

Schisandra

Schisandra chinensis, commonly known as the five-flavor berry, is a fruit-bearing vine that has been used in traditional Chinese medicine for centuries. This herb is known for its unique combination of five flavors: sour, bitter, sweet, salty, and pungent[1]. Schisandra has been traditionally used to improve vitality, enhance physical performance, and protect the liver. Recent studies have also suggested that Schisandra may have beneficial effects on diabetes and blood sugar management[2].

Active Ingredients and Compounds

Schisandra contains a variety of active ingredients, including **lignans** (such as schisandrin A, B, and C), **triterpenoids**, **flavonoids**, and organic acids. These compounds are believed to contribute to its antioxidant, anti-inflammatory, and **adaptogenic** properties[3]. Lignans, in particular, have been shown to improve insulin sensitivity and protect beta cells in the pancreas, which are crucial for maintaining normal blood sugar levels.

Mechanism of Action

The exact mechanism of action of Schisandra in managing diabetes and blood sugar is not fully understood. However, studies suggest that its antioxidant and anti-inflammatory properties play a significant role[3]. Schisandra may help reduce oxidative stress and inflammation, which are common factors in the development of diabetes. Additionally, its adaptogenic properties help the body adapt to stress, which can also contribute to better blood sugar control[5].

History of Use

Schisandra has a long history of use in traditional Chinese medicine, dating back over 2,000 years. It was used by Taoist monks to enhance their spiritual practices and by hunters to improve their endurance and **night vision**[2]. In Russia, Schisandra was recognized as an adaptogen in the 1960s, and it has been used to **combat fatigue and improve physical performance**.

Doses

The optimal dose of Schisandra for diabetes and blood sugar management has not been established. However, typical doses range from 1.5 to 6 grams of dried fruit per day, or 300 to 600 milligrams of standardized extract[6]. It is important to consult with a healthcare provider before starting any new supplement, especially if you have underlying health conditions.

Types and How to Supplement

Schisandra is available in various forms, including dried fruit, capsules, tinctures, and teas. Dried fruit can be consumed directly or brewed into a tea, while capsules and tinctures offer a more convenient way to take standardized doses6. It is important to choose a high-quality supplement from a reputable source to ensure purity and potency.

Conclusion

Schisandra is a promising herb with potential benefits for diabetes and blood sugar management. Its active ingredients, antioxidant and anti-inflammatory properties, and adaptogenic effects make it a valuable addition to a holistic approach to health. However, more research is needed to fully understand its mechanisms and establish optimal dosing guidelines.

Sumac

Sumac (Rhus coriaria) is a spice commonly used in Middle Eastern cuisine, known for its tangy flavor and vibrant red color. Beyond its culinary uses, sumac has been studied for its potential health benefits, including its effects on diabetes.

Compounds Derived from Sumac

- **Flavonoids**: Sumac is rich in flavonoids, which are known for their antioxidant properties. These compounds help in reducing oxidative stress, a significant factor in the development of diabetes[1].
- **Tannins**: These polyphenolic compounds have anti-inflammatory and antioxidant effects, contributing to the overall health benefits of sumac[1].
- **Organic Acids**: Sumac contains various organic acids, such as malic acid and citric acid, which contribute to its antioxidant capacity[2].
- **Phenolic Compounds**: These compounds, including gallic acid and methyl gallate, have been shown to exhibit antidiabetic properties by modulating glucose metabolism[2].

Mechanisms of Action

- **Antioxidant Properties**: The high content of flavonoids and phenolic compounds in sumac helps in scavenging free radicals and reducing oxidative stress. This is crucial in managing diabetes, as oxidative stress can damage pancreatic beta cells and impair insulin secretion[1].
- **Anti-inflammatory Effects**: Sumac reduces inflammation by inhibiting the production of pro-inflammatory cytokines. Chronic inflammation is a known contributor to insulin resistance and the progression of diabetes[2].
- **Inhibition of Carbohydrate-Digesting Enzymes**: Sumac has been shown to inhibit the activity of α-amylase and α-glucosidase, enzymes involved in the breakdown of carbohydrates. This inhibition slows down the absorption of glucose, leading to lower postprandial blood glucose levels[3].
- **Improvement of Lipid Profiles**: Sumac improves lipid profiles by reducing total cholesterol, LDL cholesterol, and triglycerides, which

are often elevated in diabetic patients. This contributes to better cardiovascular health[4].

Effects on Diabetes

- **Reduction of Blood Glucose Levels**: Sumac has been shown to significantly lower fasting blood glucose levels and improve glycemic control. This is achieved through its antioxidant, anti-inflammatory, and enzyme-inhibiting properties[3].
- **Improved Insulin Sensitivity**: By reducing oxidative stress and inflammation, sumac helps improve insulin sensitivity, which is crucial for effective glucose metabolism[2].
- **Cardiovascular Benefits**: The improvement in lipid profiles and reduction in oxidative stress contribute to better cardiovascular health, reducing the risk of complications associated with diabetes[4].
- **Protection Against Diabetic Complications**: Sumac's antioxidant and anti-inflammatory properties help protect against complications such as diabetic neuropathy, nephropathy, and retinopathy[1].

Dosages

The optimal dosage of sumac for managing diabetes varies, but studies suggest that doses ranging from **500 to 1000 mg per day** are generally safe and effective[4]. It is advisable to start with a lower dose and gradually increase it to monitor tolerance and effectiveness. Consulting with a healthcare provider before starting supplementation is recommended to tailor the dosage to individual needs and conditions[4].

Conclusion

Sumac, through its antioxidant, anti-inflammatory, and enzyme-inhibiting properties, offers significant therapeutic benefits for diabetes. Its mechanisms of action contribute to improved glycemic control, better lipid profiles, and protection against diabetic complications. While more research is needed to establish optimal dosages and long-term safety, current evidence supports the potential of sumac as a valuable supplement in managing diabetes.

THC Marijuana

Tetrahydrocannabinol (THC) is the primary psychoactive compound found in marijuana. While marijuana has been used for various medicinal purposes, its effects on blood sugar and diabetes management are complex and still under investigation.

Mechanisms of Action

- **Improving Insulin Sensitivity**: Some studies suggest that THC may help improve insulin sensitivity. Research has shown that marijuana users tend to have lower fasting insulin levels and a lower likelihood of insulin resistance compared to non-users[1]. Improved insulin sensitivity means that the body can use insulin more effectively to lower blood sugar levels.
- **Regulating Blood Sugar Levels**: THC may help regulate blood sugar levels by influencing the endocannabinoid system, which plays a role in energy balance and glucose metabolism[2]. Some studies have found that THC can lower fasting blood glucose levels and improve pancreatic beta-cell function, which is crucial for insulin production[3].
- **Managing Weight and Appetite**: Weight management is an important aspect of diabetes control. Some research indicates that marijuana users tend to have a smaller waist circumference and lower body mass index (BMI) compared to non-users[4]. However, THC is also known to increase appetite, which can lead to higher calorie intake and potential weight gain. This effect, often referred to as the "munchies," can be a double-edged sword for individuals with diabetes.
- **Reducing Inflammation and Neuropathy**: Chronic inflammation and neuropathy (nerve damage) are common complications of diabetes. THC has anti-inflammatory properties that may help reduce inflammation and alleviate pain associated with diabetic neuropathy[1]. This can improve the quality of life for individuals suffering from these complications.

Clinical Evidence

The clinical evidence on THC marijuana and diabetes is still emerging. A study published in Diabetes Care found that marijuana use was associated with lower fasting insulin levels and improved insulin sensitivity[1]. Another study highlighted that THC significantly decreased fasting blood glucose levels and improved pancreatic beta-cell function in people with type 2 diabetes[3]. However, it is important to note that the research is not entirely conclusive. Some studies have reported mixed results, and there is a need for more extensive clinical trials to fully understand the long-term effects of THC on blood sugar and diabetes management[2].

Dosage and Safety

The dosage of THC can vary widely depending on the form of marijuana used (e.g., smoking, edibles, tinctures) and individual tolerance. It is crucial to start with a low dose and gradually increase it under the guidance of a healthcare provider. THC can cause side effects such as dizziness, dry mouth, and altered mental state, which can affect daily functioning[1]. Additionally, marijuana use is still illegal in many places, and its legal status should be considered.

Conclusion

THC marijuana offers potential benefits for managing blood sugar and diabetes, particularly in improving insulin sensitivity, regulating blood sugar levels, and reducing inflammation. However, its effects can vary, and more research is needed to fully understand its long-term impact. As always, it is essential to discuss any new treatments or supplements with a healthcare provider to ensure they are safe and appropriate for individual health needs.

Turmeric

Turmeric, a golden-yellow spice derived from the root of the Curcuma longa plant, has been used for centuries in traditional medicine. Its active component, curcumin, is credited with numerous health benefits, including potential effects on blood sugar control and diabetes management.

Mechanisms of Action

- **Improving Insulin Sensitivity**: Curcumin has been shown to enhance insulin sensitivity, which is crucial for managing type 2 diabetes. It activates AMP-activated protein kinase (AMPK), an enzyme that plays a key role in cellular energy homeostasis. By activating AMPK, curcumin helps improve the body's response to insulin, facilitating better glucose uptake by cells and lowering blood sugar levels[1].
- **Regulating Blood Sugar Levels**: Curcumin helps regulate blood sugar levels by influencing the activity of enzymes involved in glucose metabolism. It can decrease the production of glucose in the liver and increase glucose uptake in muscle cells[2]. This dual action helps maintain stable blood sugar levels and prevents hyperglycemia.
- **Anti-inflammatory and Antioxidant Properties**: Chronic inflammation and oxidative stress are significant contributors to the development and progression of diabetes. Curcumin's potent anti-inflammatory and antioxidant properties help reduce inflammation and protect cells from oxidative damage[3]. This can improve overall metabolic health and prevent complications such as cardiovascular disease.

Clinical Evidence

Several studies have demonstrated the efficacy of curcumin in managing diabetes. For instance, a systematic review published in Frontiers in Endocrinology highlighted that curcumin significantly reduces fasting blood glucose, glycated hemoglobin (HbA1c), and body mass index (BMI) in individuals with diabetes[4]. Another study found that curcumin supplementation improved insulin sensitivity and reduced fasting blood glucose levels in people with type 2 diabetes[5].

A 2021 review of studies suggested that curcumin can decrease blood sugar levels and reduce diabetes-related complications[1]. The researchers noted that curcumin might also play a role in diabetes prevention by improving insulin sensitivity and reducing inflammation.

Dosage and Safety

The typical dosage of curcumin used in studies ranges from 500 to 2,000 mg per day, usually in the form of standardized extracts. It is generally well-tolerated, but some individuals may experience mild side effects such as gastrointestinal discomfort or nausea[6]. It is important to consult with a healthcare provider before starting curcumin supplementation, especially for individuals taking other medications, as curcumin can interact with certain drugs.

Conclusion

Turmeric, through its active component curcumin, offers several potential benefits for managing diabetes, particularly in improving insulin sensitivity, regulating blood sugar levels, and reducing inflammation and oxidative stress. While it is not a replacement for conventional diabetes treatments, turmeric can be a valuable addition to a comprehensive diabetes management plan. As always, it is essential to discuss any new supplements with a healthcare provider to ensure they are safe and appropriate for individual health needs.

Vanadium

Vanadium is a trace mineral found in various foods, including mushrooms, shellfish, black pepper, and grains. It has garnered attention for its potential benefits in managing diabetes, particularly type 2 diabetes. Although research is still ongoing, several studies have highlighted vanadium's insulin-mimetic properties and its role in glucose metabolism. This one is one I would recommend adding to your daily stack.

Mechanisms of Action

- **Insulin-Mimetic Properties**: Vanadium compounds, such as vanadyl sulfate and sodium metavanadate, have been shown to mimic the effects of insulin. These compounds can activate insulin receptors and enhance the signaling pathways involved in glucose uptake[1]. This insulin-like activity helps lower blood sugar levels by promoting glucose transport into cells, similar to the action of insulin.
- **Improving Glucose Metabolism**: Vanadium has been found to improve glucose metabolism by enhancing the activity of enzymes involved in glucose oxidation and glycogen synthesis[2]. This helps the body utilize glucose more efficiently, reducing blood sugar levels and improving overall metabolic control.
- **Reducing Insulin Resistance**: Insulin resistance is a key feature of type 2 diabetes, where the body's cells become less responsive to insulin. Vanadium compounds have been shown to reduce insulin resistance by improving the sensitivity of insulin receptors[3]. This leads to better glucose uptake and utilization, helping to maintain stable blood sugar levels.

Clinical Evidence

Several studies have investigated the effects of vanadium on diabetes management. For example, a study published in Diabetes Care found that vanadyl sulfate supplementation improved insulin sensitivity and reduced fasting blood glucose levels in people with type 2 diabetes[4]. Another study highlighted that vanadium compounds lowered HbA1c levels, a marker of long-term blood sugar control, in diabetic patients[5].

Dosage and Safety

The typical dosage of vanadium used in studies ranges from 50 to 100 mg per day, usually in the form of vanadyl sulfate. However, it is important to note that high doses of vanadium can be toxic and may cause side effects such as gastrointestinal discomfort, nausea, and diarrhea[6]. Long-term use of high doses can also lead to more serious health issues, including kidney and liver damage. Therefore, it is crucial to consult with a healthcare provider before starting vanadium supplementation, especially for individuals with pre-existing health conditions.

Conclusion

Vanadium offers several potential benefits for people with diabetes, particularly in mimicking insulin, improving glucose metabolism, and reducing insulin resistance. While it is not a replacement for conventional diabetes treatments, vanadium can be a valuable addition to a comprehensive diabetes management plan. As always, it is essential to discuss any new supplements with a healthcare provider to ensure they are safe and appropriate for individual health needs.

Vitamin B8 (Inositol)

Vitamin B8, more commonly known as **inositol**, is a naturally occurring compound that plays a crucial role in various biological processes within the body. Although not officially classified as a vitamin, inositol is often grouped with the B-vitamin complex due to its importance in cell function and growth. In recent years, inositol has gained attention for its potential benefits in managing diabetes, particularly Type 2 diabetes and its associated conditions like insulin resistance and metabolic syndrome.

History of Inositol

Inositol was first isolated in 1850 by the German chemist Johann Joseph Scherer from muscle tissue, hence its initial name "muscle sugar." The term "inositol" derives from the Greek word *inos*, meaning "muscle." It wasn't until later that inositol was found to be widespread in plants and animals, including humans. Initially considered a vitamin (vitamin B8), it was later reclassified since the human body can synthesize inositol from glucose. However, certain conditions may increase the body's demand for inositol beyond what it can produce, making dietary intake or supplementation beneficial.

Inositol's Effects on Diabetes

Inositol plays a critical role in cellular signaling pathways, particularly those involving insulin. It exists in nine stereoisomeric forms, with myo-inositol and D-chiro-inositol being the most biologically significant. These two forms are involved in the insulin signaling cascade:

- **Insulin Signal Transduction**: Inositol phosphoglycans (IPGs) derived from myo-inositol and D-chiro-inositol act as secondary messengers in insulin signal transduction. They facilitate glucose uptake by enhancing the activity of glucose transporter proteins (GLUT4) on cell membranes.

- **Improving Insulin Sensitivity**: Myo-inositol and D-chiro-inositol improve insulin sensitivity by promoting the efficient use of insulin and reducing insulin resistance, a hallmark of Type 2 diabetes.

- **Regulating Glucose Metabolism**: Inositol compounds help regulate enzymes involved in glucose metabolism, such as glycogen synthase and pyruvate dehydrogenase, thus enhancing glucose utilization and storage.

How Inositol Helps in Diabetes Management

- **Reducing Insulin Resistance**: By improving insulin signal transduction, inositol enhances the body's response to insulin, allowing for better blood glucose control.

- **Lowering Blood Glucose Levels**: Improved insulin sensitivity leads to more efficient glucose uptake by cells, reducing hyperglycemia.

- **Enhancing Ovarian Function in PCOS**: In women with polycystic ovary syndrome (PCOS), a condition often associated with insulin resistance, inositol supplementation has been shown to restore ovulation and improve fertility.

- **Antioxidant Properties**: Inositol exhibits antioxidant effects that may protect pancreatic β-cells from oxidative stress-induced damage, preserving insulin secretion capacity.

- **Supporting Lipid Metabolism**: It aids in reducing triglyceride and cholesterol levels, thereby improving lipid profiles commonly disturbed in diabetic patients.

Types of Inositol Supplementation

- **Myo-Inositol (MI):** The most abundant form in nature and the human body, primarily used for improving insulin sensitivity and ovarian function in PCOS.

- **D-Chiro-Inositol (DCI):** Formed from myo-inositol via insulin-dependent epimerase enzymes; effective in reducing insulin resistance and hyperandrogenism.

- **Combined MI and DCI Supplements**: Evidence suggests that a combination of both, in a physiological ratio (typically 40:1 of MI to DCI), provides synergistic benefits for insulin sensitivity and endocrine function.

- **Inositol Hexaphosphate (IP6)**: Also known as phytic acid, found in high-fiber foods; has antioxidant properties but less studied in the context of diabetes.

Recommended Doses

- For Insulin Resistance and Type 2 Diabetes:

    - **Myo-Inositol**: Typically, doses range from 2 grams twice daily (total of 4 grams per day).

    - **D-Chiro-Inositol**: Doses of 500 mg to 1 gram per day are common.

    - **Combined MI/DCI Supplements**: Often provided in a 40:1 ratio, matching physiological plasma ratios, e.g., 2000 mg MI with 50 mg DCI twice daily.

- **For PCOS Management**:

    - Similar dosing as above, with studies often using 4 grams of myo-inositol per day, sometimes in combination with folic acid.

Note: It is important to consult a healthcare provider before starting supplementation to determine the appropriate dosage and ensure safety, especially for individuals with existing medical conditions or those taking other medications.

Scientific Evidence and Studies

- **Pacioni et al., 2020**: Demonstrated that myo-inositol supplementation improves insulin sensitivity and reduces fasting glucose levels in patients with Type 2 diabetes.

- **D'Anna et al., 2017**: Found that combined myo-inositol and D-chiro-inositol supplementation improved metabolic and hormonal parameters in women with gestational diabetes.

- **Laganà et al., 2018**: Reported that inositol supplementation enhanced ovarian function and metabolic profiles in women with PCOS, reducing insulin resistance.

Conclusion

Inositol (vitamin B8) plays a significant role in the management of diabetes through its impact on insulin signaling pathways and glucose metabolism. Its ability to enhance insulin sensitivity and lower blood glucose levels makes it a valuable adjunct therapy in Type 2 diabetes management. Supplementation with myo-inositol, D-chiro-inositol, or a combination of both has been shown to provide metabolic benefits, particularly in individuals with insulin resistance or PCOS-related insulin dysregulation. While generally considered safe, it is advisable to consult healthcare professionals for personalized dosing and to evaluate potential interactions with other treatments.

Vitamin D

Vitamin D, often referred to as the "sunshine vitamin," is a fat-soluble vitamin that plays a crucial role in maintaining bone health, immune function, and overall well-being. Recent research has also highlighted its potential impact on blood sugar regulation and diabetes management[2]. Vitamin D has been used for centuries to treat rickets; a bone disease caused by vitamin D deficiency. In the early 20th century, the discovery of vitamin D and its role in bone health led to the fortification of foods with vitamin D, significantly reducing the incidence of rickets[1]. Today, vitamin D supplements are widely used to address deficiencies and support overall health.

Vitamin D and Blood Sugar Regulation

Vitamin D is believed to **improve the body's sensitivity to insulin**, the hormone responsible for regulating blood sugar levels. Studies have shown that individuals with low vitamin D levels are more likely to develop insulin resistance, a precursor to type 2 diabetes[2]. Vitamin D deficiency has also been linked to higher levels of inflammatory markers and **impaired pancreatic beta-cell function**, both of which can contribute to the development of diabetes.

Vitamin D and Diabetes Management

Research suggests that vitamin D supplementation may help manage type 2 diabetes. A study involving adults at high risk for diabetes found that those who took vitamin D supplements were 12% less likely to develop diabetes compared to those who received a placebo[2]. However, the results were not statistically significant, and more research is needed to establish a definitive link.

Vitamin D2 vs. D3

Vitamin D exists in two main forms: vitamin **D2 (ergocalciferol)** and vitamin **D3 (cholecalciferol)**. Vitamin D3 is synthesized from sun exposure and can be ingested through food and supplements, while vitamin D2 is primarily obtained from plant sources and fortified foods4. Studies suggest that vitamin

D3 is more effective at raising blood levels of vitamin D compared to vitamin D2.

Compounds and Mechanism of Action

Vitamin D2 and D3 are converted into their active form, calcitriol, in the liver and kidneys. Calcitriol then binds to vitamin D receptors in various tissues, including the pancreas, where it helps regulate insulin secretion and sensitivity[2].

Recommended Doses

The recommended daily intake of vitamin D varies based on age, sex, and health status. For most adults, the recommended dietary allowance (RDA) is 600-800 IU (15-20 mcg) per day[1]. However, some studies suggest that higher doses may be needed to achieve optimal blood levels, especially for individuals with diabetes or at risk of deficiency.

Sunshine Requirement

The amount of sunshine needed to produce sufficient vitamin D varies based on factors such as skin color, geographic location, and time of year. Generally, it is recommended to get 10-30 minutes of midday sun exposure several times a week, with hands, face, and arms exposed[1]. However, individuals with darker skin or living in northern latitudes may need more sun exposure or consider vitamin D supplementation.

Conclusion

Vitamin D plays a vital role in blood sugar regulation and diabetes management. While more research is needed to establish definitive links, maintaining adequate vitamin D levels through sun exposure, diet, and supplements can contribute to overall health and well-being.

White Mulberry

White mulberry (Morus alba) is a deciduous tree native to China, known for its white-colored fruit and medicinal properties. It has been traditionally used in Chinese medicine for various health conditions, including diabetes[2]. Recent studies have shown that white mulberry can help manage blood sugar levels, making it a potential natural remedy for diabetes.

Active Ingredients and Compounds

White mulberry contains several bioactive compounds, including **flavonoids**, **phenolic acids**, **terpenoids**, and **alkaloids**. The primary active ingredients responsible for its antidiabetic effects are **1-deoxynojirimycin (DNJ)**, **fagomine**, and **N-methyl-1-deoxynojirimycin**. These compounds inhibit alpha-glucosidase, an enzyme that breaks down carbohydrates into glucose, thereby reducing postprandial blood sugar levels[4].

Mechanism of Action

The mechanism of action of white mulberry involves the inhibition of carbohydrate digestion and absorption. By inhibiting alpha-glucosidase, DNJ and other active compounds slow down the breakdown of complex carbohydrates into simple sugars, preventing rapid spikes in blood glucose levels[4]. This helps maintain stable blood sugar levels and improves insulin sensitivity.

History of Use

White mulberry has a long history of use in traditional Chinese medicine, dating back to AD 659. It has been used to treat various conditions, including diabetes, high cholesterol, and high blood pressure[1]. The leaves, roots, and fruits of the white mulberry tree have been documented in the Pharmacopoeia of the People's Republic of China for their medicinal properties.

Doses

The typical dose of white mulberry leaf powder or extract for managing diabetes is **0.8-1 gram three times daily** before meals. It is important to consult a healthcare provider before starting any supplement to determine the appropriate dosage for individual needs[1].

Types and How to Supplement

White mulberry is available in various forms, including leaf powder, capsules, and extracts. It can be taken as a supplement or added to foods and beverages. When choosing a supplement, look for third-party tested products to ensure quality and safety[5]. Always follow the manufacturer's instructions for dosage and consult a healthcare provider if you have any underlying health conditions or are taking other medications.

Conclusion

White mulberry shows promise as a natural remedy for managing diabetes and blood sugar levels. Its active compounds, particularly DNJ, help slow carbohydrate digestion and absorption, leading to more stable blood glucose levels4. However, more research is needed to fully understand its effects and establish standardized dosages. As with any supplement, it is essential to consult a healthcare provider before use.

Wormwood

Wormwood, scientifically known as Artemisia absinthium, is a perennial herb with a rich history of use in traditional medicine. Wormwood has been used by various Native American tribes for its medicinal properties. Known for its bitter taste and potent aroma, wormwood was often employed to treat digestive issues, fevers, and parasitic infections[1]. The plant, referred to as tl'ogh tsen in the Ahtna language, was also used in spiritual practices, such as smudging to ward off negative energy[1].

In Alaska, Indigenous peoples like the St. Lawrence Island Yupik have utilized wormwood for its healing properties. It was used in salves for aches and pains, teas for respiratory ailments, and as a smudge to cleanse spaces[1]. This deep-rooted knowledge of wormwood's benefits has been passed down through generations, highlighting its importance in Native American herbal medicine.

Effects on Blood Sugar and Diabetes

Recent research has begun to explore the potential benefits of wormwood in managing blood sugar levels and diabetes. Here are some key findings:

- **Blood Sugar Regulation**: Studies suggest that wormwood may help balance blood sugar levels and improve insulin sensitivity. This is particularly beneficial for individuals with type 2 diabetes, as it can help manage blood sugar spikes and improve overall glycemic control[2].
- **Anti-Inflammatory Properties**: Wormwood contains compounds with anti-inflammatory effects, which can help reduce inflammation associated with diabetes[2]. Chronic inflammation is a known contributor to insulin resistance and type 2 diabetes.
- **Lipid Metabolism**: Wormwood may also prevent the accumulation of lipids in the blood, which is crucial for individuals with diabetes who are at higher risk of cardiovascular diseases[2]. By improving lipid metabolism, wormwood can support overall metabolic health.
- **Antioxidant Effects**: The herb is rich in antioxidants, which help protect cells from oxidative stress and damage. This is particularly important for individuals with diabetes, as oxidative stress can exacerbate complications associated with the disease[2].

Considerations and Precautions

While wormwood shows promise in managing blood sugar levels and supporting diabetes treatment, it is important to use it under professional guidance. Wormwood contains thujone, a compound that can be toxic in high doses[2]. Therefore, it is crucial to adhere to recommended dosages and consult with a healthcare provider before incorporating wormwood into a diabetes management plan.

Conclusion

Wormwood has a long history of use in Native American medicine for its healing properties. Recent research suggests that it may also offer benefits for managing blood sugar levels and diabetes. However, due to its potent compounds, it should be used with caution and under professional supervision. Understanding the traditional and modern uses of wormwood can help us appreciate its potential as a natural remedy for diabetes and other health conditions.

Neuropathy

Neuropathy and Its Connection to Diabetes

Neuropathy, a condition characterized by nerve damage, is a common complication of diabetes. Diabetic neuropathy, specifically, refers to nerve damage caused by prolonged high blood sugar levels[1]. This condition can affect various parts of the body, including the peripheral nerves, autonomic nerves, and proximal nerves.

Causes of Neuropathy

Neuropathy can result from several factors, including:

- **Diabetes**: High blood sugar levels can damage blood vessels that supply nerves, leading to neuropathy.
- **Vitamin Deficiencies**: Lack of essential vitamins, particularly B vitamins, can contribute to nerve damage.
- **Autoimmune Diseases**: Conditions like rheumatoid arthritis can cause neuropathy.
- **Infections**: Certain infections, such as HIV/AIDS and leprosy, can lead to neuropathy.
- **Injuries**: Trauma or physical injury to nerves can result in neuropathy.
- **Genetic Disorders**: Conditions like Friedreich's ataxia can cause neuropathy.
- **Toxins**: Exposure to toxins, including certain medications and chemotherapy drugs, can damage nerves.

Blood Sugar Correlation

High blood sugar levels are a significant risk factor for neuropathy. **Prolonged hyperglycemia can lead to metabolic disturbances that damage nerve fibers**[3]. Studies have shown that maintaining blood glucose levels within the target range can help prevent or delay the onset of neuropathy.

Damage to the Myelin Sheath

The myelin sheath, a protective covering around nerve fibers, can be damaged by high blood sugar levels. This damage disrupts the transmission of nerve signals, leading to symptoms such as numbness, tingling, and pain[1]. Over time, the loss of myelin can result in muscle weakness and loss of coordination.

Scientific Studies

Recent studies have explored the mechanisms underlying diabetic neuropathy. For example, a study published in Diabetes, Metabolic Syndrome and Obesity found that lower levels of free triiodothyronine (FT3) were associated with an increased risk of diabetic peripheral neuropathy in patients with type 2 diabetes. The study highlighted the importance of thyroid hormones in nerve health and suggested that monitoring FT3 levels could help in managing neuropathy[6].

Treatment and Management

Managing neuropathy involves a combination of lifestyle changes, medications, and therapies. Key strategies include:

- **Blood Sugar Control**: Keeping blood glucose levels within the target range is crucial for preventing further nerve damage.
- **Medications**: Pain relievers, anti-seizure medications, and antidepressants can help manage neuropathy symptoms.
- **Therapies**: Physical therapy, occupational therapy, and transcutaneous electrical nerve stimulation (TENS) can improve nerve function and reduce pain.
- **Lifestyle Changes**: Regular exercise, a healthy diet, and avoiding alcohol can support nerve health.

The Myelin Sheath

The myelin sheath is a critical component of the nervous system, playing a vital role in the efficient transmission of electrical impulses along nerve cells. In the previous chapter it talks about damage to the myelin sheath, knowing and understanding what the myelin sheath is made of, gives us a way to repair and fix the damaged caused by the high blood sugar.

Composition of the Myelin Sheath

The myelin sheath is primarily composed of lipids (fats) and proteins, forming a protective, insulating layer around the axons of nerve cells. The key components include:

- **Lipids**: Myelin is rich in lipids, which make up about 70-80% of its dry weight. The primary lipid components are phospholipids, cholesterol, and glycolipids. These lipids provide the insulating properties necessary for the myelin sheath to function effectively[1].
- **Proteins**: The remaining 20-30% of the myelin sheath is composed of proteins. The major proteins include myelin basic protein (MBP) and proteolipid protein (PLP). These proteins help maintain the structural integrity of the myelin sheath and facilitate its formation and maintenance[2].
- **Glial Cells**: Myelin is produced by specialized glial cells. In the central nervous system (CNS), oligodendrocytes are responsible for myelination, while in the peripheral nervous system (PNS), Schwann cells perform this function[3].

Function of the Myelin Sheath

The myelin sheath serves several crucial functions in the nervous system:

- **Insulation**: The primary function of the myelin sheath is to insulate nerve fibers. This insulation prevents the loss of electrical signals as they travel along the axon, much like the plastic coating around electrical wires[1].
- **Increased Conduction Speed**: Myelin significantly increases the speed at which electrical impulses (action potentials) travel along the axon. This is achieved through a process called saltatory conduction, where the electrical impulse jumps from one node of Ranvier (gaps in

the myelin sheath) to the next, rather than traveling continuously along the axon[2].

- **Protection and Maintenance**: The myelin sheath protects nerve fibers from physical damage and helps maintain the strength and integrity of the electrical signals as they travel along the axon[1].
- **Energy Efficiency**: By enabling faster signal transmission, the myelin sheath reduces the energy required for nerve cells to transmit impulses. This efficiency is crucial for the proper functioning of the nervous system[4].

Importance of the Myelin Sheath

The myelin sheath is essential for the proper functioning of the nervous system. Damage to the myelin sheath can lead to a range of neurological disorders, including multiple sclerosis (MS) and Guillain-Barré syndrome. In these conditions, the loss of myelin disrupts the efficient transmission of electrical signals, leading to symptoms such as muscle weakness, coordination problems, and sensory disturbances[2].

Conclusion

The myelin sheath, composed of lipids and proteins, is a vital structure that insulates nerve fibers, increases conduction speed, protects nerve cells, and enhances energy efficiency. Its role in maintaining the integrity and speed of electrical signal transmission is crucial for the proper functioning of the nervous system. Understanding the composition and function of the myelin sheath underscores its importance in health and disease, highlighting the need for ongoing research to protect, repair, and regenerate this essential component of the nervous system.

Acetyl-L-Carnitine (ALC)

Acetyl-L-carnitine (ALC) is a naturally occurring compound that has garnered attention for its potential benefits in managing neuropathy. ALC is an acetylated form of L-carnitine, an amino acid derivative that plays a crucial role in energy production. It is involved in the transport of fatty acids into the mitochondria, where they are oxidized to produce energy[1]. ALC is both water- and fat-soluble, allowing it to cross the blood-brain barrier and exert effects on the central nervous system[1].

Effects on Neuropathy

Neuropathy, particularly peripheral neuropathy, involves damage to the peripheral nerves, leading to symptoms such as pain, tingling, and numbness. ALC has shown promise in alleviating these symptoms through several mechanisms:

- **Pain Reduction**: Clinical studies have demonstrated that ALC can significantly reduce neuropathic pain. It helps alleviate symptoms by reducing oxidative stress and inflammation, which are key contributors to nerve damage[2].
- **Improved Nerve Function**: ALC has been shown to improve nerve conduction and function. This is particularly beneficial for individuals with diabetic neuropathy, as it helps restore normal nerve activity[2].
- **Neuroprotection**: ALC provides neuroprotective effects by safeguarding nerve cells from further damage. This is achieved through its antioxidant properties, which help reduce oxidative stress and inflammation[2].
- **Nerve Regeneration**: ALC promotes the regeneration of nerve fibers, enhancing the repair of damaged nerves and improving overall nerve function[2].

Active Compounds and Mechanisms of Action

The beneficial effects of ALC on neuropathy are primarily attributed to its role in energy metabolism and its antioxidant properties. Here's how ALC and its related compounds work:

- **Energy Metabolism**: ALC facilitates the transport of fatty acids into the mitochondria, where they are converted into energy. This process is crucial for maintaining the health and function of nerve cells[1].
- **Antioxidant Properties**: ALC acts as a powerful antioxidant, neutralizing free radicals that cause oxidative stress. It also regenerates other antioxidants, such as vitamins C and E, enhancing the body's overall antioxidant defense system[3]. This helps protect nerve cells from damage and supports their repair.
- **Anti-Inflammatory Effects**: ALC reduces inflammation by inhibiting the activation of nuclear factor-kappa B (NF-κB), a protein complex that plays a key role in regulating the immune response to inflammation[3]. By reducing inflammation, ALC helps alleviate pain and prevent further nerve damage.
- **Neurotrophic Activity**: ALC increases levels of nerve growth factor (NGF), which supports the growth, maintenance, and survival of neurons[2]. This neurotrophic activity is essential for nerve regeneration and repair.
- **Improved Blood Flow**: ALC improves microcirculation, which is crucial for delivering nutrients and oxygen to nerve cells. Enhanced blood flow helps support nerve health and function[4].

Conclusion

Acetyl-L-carnitine (ALC) is a versatile compound with significant potential benefits for managing neuropathy. Its role in energy metabolism, antioxidant and anti-inflammatory properties, and ability to promote nerve regeneration make it a valuable supplement for individuals suffering from neuropathic pain. However, it is important to use ALC under the guidance of a healthcare professional to ensure safety and efficacy.

Alpha-Lipoic Acid (ALA)

Alpha-lipoic acid (ALA) is a naturally occurring compound that has gained attention for its potential benefits in managing neuropathy.

What is Alpha-Lipoic Acid (ALA)?

ALA is a fatty acid found in every cell of the body, where it helps convert glucose into energy. It is both water- and fat-soluble, allowing it to work in every part of the cell[1]. ALA is also a powerful antioxidant, which means it can neutralize harmful free radicals that cause oxidative stress and damage cells[1].

Effects on Neuropathy

Neuropathy, particularly diabetic neuropathy, involves damage to the peripheral nerves, leading to symptoms such as pain, tingling, and numbness. ALA has shown promise in alleviating these symptoms through several mechanisms:

- **Pain Reduction**: Clinical studies have demonstrated that ALA can significantly reduce neuropathic pain. It helps alleviate symptoms by reducing oxidative stress and inflammation, which are key contributors to nerve damage[2].
- **Improved Nerve Function**: ALA has been shown to improve nerve conduction and function. This is particularly beneficial for individuals with diabetic neuropathy, as it helps restore normal nerve activity[2].
- **Neuroprotection**: ALA provides neuroprotective effects by safeguarding nerve cells from further damage. This is achieved through its antioxidant properties, which help reduce oxidative stress and inflammation[2].

Active Compounds and Mechanisms of Action

The beneficial effects of ALA on neuropathy are primarily attributed to its antioxidant and anti-inflammatory properties. Here's how ALA and its related compounds work:

- **Antioxidant Properties**: ALA acts as a powerful antioxidant, neutralizing free radicals that cause oxidative stress. It also regenerates other antioxidants, such as vitamins C and E, enhancing the body's overall antioxidant defense system[3]. This helps protect nerve cells from damage and supports their repair.

- **Anti-Inflammatory Effects**: ALA reduces inflammation by inhibiting the activation of nuclear factor-kappa B (NF-κB), a protein complex that plays a key role in regulating the immune response to inflammation[3]. By reducing inflammation, ALA helps alleviate pain and prevent further nerve damage.
- **Regeneration of Nerve Cells**: ALA promotes the regeneration of nerve cells by enhancing the production of nerve growth factors. This supports the repair and regeneration of damaged nerves, improving overall nerve function[3].
- **Improved Blood Flow**: ALA improves microcirculation, which is crucial for delivering nutrients and oxygen to nerve cells. Enhanced blood flow helps support nerve health and function[4].

Conclusion

Alpha-lipoic acid (ALA) is a versatile compound with significant potential benefits for managing neuropathy. Its antioxidant and anti-inflammatory properties, along with its ability to improve nerve function and promote nerve regeneration, make it a valuable supplement for individuals suffering from neuropathic pain. However, it is important to use ALA under the guidance of a healthcare professional to ensure safety and efficacy.

Arnica

Arnica montana, commonly known as arnica, is a perennial herb native to Europe and Siberia. Historically used for its anti-inflammatory and analgesic properties, arnica has gained attention for its potential benefits in treating neuropathic pain. Arnica has been utilized for centuries in traditional herbal medicine. Documented as early as the 16th century, it was popularly used in Europe for treating bruises, sprains, muscle aches, rheumatic pain, and inflammation. The flower heads are the primary medicinal parts of the plant, often prepared as topical ointments, creams, gels, or tinctures. In addition to its external applications, diluted homeopathic preparations of arnica have been used internally, although this practice is controversial due to potential toxicity.

Compounds and Ingredients

- Sesquiterpene Lactones: The most significant are helenalin and its derivatives, known for potent anti-inflammatory and analgesic effects.
- Flavonoids: Including quercetin, luteolin, and isoquercitrin, which have antioxidant properties.
- Phenolic Acids: Such as caffeic acid and chlorogenic acid, contributing to antioxidant activity.
- Volatile Oils: Containing thymol derivatives with antimicrobial activity.
- Polysaccharides: Which may enhance immune function.

Mechanism of Action

- Inhibition of Nuclear Factor-kappa B (NF-κB): Helenalin inhibits NF-κB activation, a transcription factor that regulates genes involved in inflammatory responses. This reduces the production of pro-inflammatory cytokines like IL-1β, TNF-α, and IL-6.
- Suppression of Cyclooxygenase-2 (COX-2) Enzyme: By inhibiting COX-2, arnica reduces the synthesis of prostaglandins, lipid compounds that mediate inflammation and pain.

- Antioxidant Activity: Flavonoids and phenolic acids scavenge free radicals, decreasing oxidative stress and protecting nerve cells from damage.
- Modulation of Immune Response: Arnica compounds may decrease the migration of immune cells to inflamed areas, reducing edema and inflammation.
- Enhancement of Microcirculation: Topical application improves blood flow to affected tissues, facilitating healing and reducing pain.

Effects on Neuropathy

While direct clinical evidence is limited, the pharmacological actions of arnica suggest potential benefits for neuropathy:

- Pain Relief: By inhibiting inflammatory mediators and reducing oxidative stress, arnica may alleviate neuropathic pain.
- Nerve Protection: Antioxidant properties protect neurons from damage caused by free radicals.
- Improved Blood Flow: Enhanced microcirculation may support nerve repair and function.
- Edema Reduction: Decreasing swelling around nerves can relieve pressure and alleviate symptoms.

A study by Leu et al. (2010) demonstrated that topical arnica significantly reduced bruising and inflammation, indicating its potential in managing conditions involving inflammation and tissue damage.

Doses and Administration

Arnica is **mainly used topically** due to toxicity concerns with internal use:

- Topical Preparations: Available in creams, gels, ointments, and oils with concentrations typically ranging from 10% to 25% *Arnica montana* tincture.
  - Application: Apply a thin layer to the affected area 2-3 times daily. Avoid applying to broken skin or open wounds.
- Homeopathic Formulations: Arnica is used in highly diluted forms (e.g., 6C, 30C potencies) for internal use.
  - Dosage: Follow the manufacturer's instructions or consult a qualified homeopathic practitioner.
- Safety Precautions:

- Avoid Oral Use of Undiluted Arnica: Ingesting arnica in its raw form can cause severe side effects, including gastrointestinal distress, cardiac arrhythmias, and organ failure.
- Allergy Considerations: Individuals allergic to the Asteraceae family (e.g., daisies, marigolds) may experience allergic reactions.

Conclusion

Arnica possesses several pharmacologically active compounds that confer anti-inflammatory, analgesic, and antioxidant effects. These properties suggest that arnica may be beneficial in managing neuropathic pain and supporting nerve health. However, due to limited clinical studies specifically addressing neuropathy, more research is needed to substantiate its efficacy. As with any herbal remedy, it is essential to use arnica responsibly, adhering to recommended doses and being mindful of potential side effects. Consulting healthcare professionals before initiating treatment is advisable to ensure safety and appropriateness.

Bearberry

Bearberry, also known as Arctostaphylos uva-ursi or uva ursi, is an evergreen shrub native to the alpine forests of North America, Europe, and Asia. Traditionally used by indigenous people for its medicinal properties, bearberry has been studied for its potential benefits in treating various conditions, including neuropathy[1]. Bearberry has a long history of use in traditional medicine. Indigenous people in North America used bearberry leaves to treat urinary tract infections and other ailments[1]. Over time, its use has expanded to include treatments for bronchitis, cystitis, and enlarged prostate.

Compounds and Ingredients

The primary active compounds in bearberry are **arbutin**, **tannins**, and **hydroquinone**. Arbutin is a glycoside that inhibits tyrosinase, an enzyme responsible for melanin production, making it useful in skin-lightening treatments[2]. Tannins have astringent properties, while hydroquinone has antimicrobial effects.

Mechanism of Action

Bearberry's mechanism of action in treating neuropathy is not well-documented, but its anti-inflammatory and antioxidant properties may play a role[3]. The anti-inflammatory effects can help reduce nerve inflammation, while antioxidants can protect nerve cells from oxidative stress[3].

Doses

The typical doses of bearberry vary depending on the form and intended use. For neuropathy, it is recommended to consult with a healthcare provider to determine the appropriate dosage, as excessive intake can lead to side effects such as nausea, vomiting, and liver damage[1].

Conclusion

While bearberry shows promise in treating neuropathy due to its anti-inflammatory and antioxidant properties, more research is needed to fully understand its effects and establish safe and effective dosages. Always consult with a healthcare provider before using bearberry for neuropathy or any other condition.

Benfotiamine

Benfotiamine is a fat-soluble derivative of thiamine (vitamin B1) that has shown promise in managing neuropathy.

What is Benfotiamine?

Benfotiamine is a synthetic derivative of thiamine, designed to enhance the bioavailability and absorption of vitamin B1. Unlike water-soluble thiamine, benfotiamine is fat-soluble, allowing it to be more easily absorbed by the body and cross cell membranes more effectively[1]. This property makes benfotiamine particularly useful in treating conditions like neuropathy, where efficient delivery to nerve cells is crucial.

Effects on Neuropathy

Neuropathy, particularly diabetic neuropathy, involves damage to the peripheral nerves, leading to symptoms such as pain, tingling, and numbness. Benfotiamine has shown promise in alleviating these symptoms through several mechanisms:

- **Pain Reduction**: Clinical studies have demonstrated that benfotiamine can significantly reduce neuropathic pain. It helps alleviate symptoms by reducing oxidative stress and inflammation, which are key contributors to nerve damage[2].
- **Improved Nerve Function**: Benfotiamine has been shown to improve nerve conduction and function. This is particularly beneficial for individuals with diabetic neuropathy, as it helps restore normal nerve activity[2].
- **Neuroprotection**: Benfotiamine provides neuroprotective effects by safeguarding nerve cells from further damage. This is achieved through its antioxidant properties, which help reduce oxidative stress and inflammation[2].

Active Compounds and Mechanisms of Action

The beneficial effects of benfotiamine on neuropathy are primarily attributed to its role in cellular metabolism and its neuroprotective properties. Here's how benfotiamine and its related compounds work:

- **Advanced Glycation End-Product (AGE) Inhibition**: Benfotiamine inhibits the formation of AGEs, which are harmful compounds that accumulate in the body and contribute to nerve damage and dysfunction[1]. By preventing AGE formation, benfotiamine helps protect nerves from damage.
- **Activation of Transketolase**: Benfotiamine activates the enzyme transketolase, which plays a crucial role in the pentose phosphate pathway. This pathway is essential for glucose metabolism and the production of nucleotides and NADPH, which are vital for nerve repair and regeneration[1].
- **Antioxidant Properties**: Benfotiamine acts as a powerful antioxidant, neutralizing free radicals that cause oxidative stress. It also regenerates other antioxidants, such as vitamins C and E, enhancing the body's overall antioxidant defense system[3]. This helps protect nerve cells from damage and supports their repair.
- **Anti-Inflammatory Effects**: Benfotiamine reduces inflammation by inhibiting the activation of nuclear factor-kappa B (NF-κB), a protein complex that plays a key role in regulating the immune response to inflammation[3]. By reducing inflammation, benfotiamine helps alleviate pain and prevent further nerve damage.

Conclusion

Benfotiamine is a versatile compound with significant potential benefits for managing neuropathy. Its role in inhibiting AGE formation, activating transketolase, and providing antioxidant and anti-inflammatory effects makes it a valuable supplement for individuals suffering from neuropathic pain. However, it is important to use benfotiamine under the guidance of a healthcare professional to ensure safety and efficacy.

Bitterroot

Lewisia rediviva, **commonly known as bitterroot**, is a flowering plant native to western North America. Traditionally used by Native American tribes for various medicinal purposes, bitterroot has gained attention for its potential therapeutic benefits.

Compounds and Ingredients

Bitterroot contains several bioactive compounds that may contribute to its medicinal properties:

- **Alkaloids**: Bitterroot is known to contain alkaloids, which are nitrogen-containing compounds that can have physiological effects on humans (Moerman, 1998).
- **Glycosides**: These are compounds that can influence heart rate and have anti-inflammatory properties (Chevallier, 1996).
- **Bitter Principles**: The plant contains bitter-tasting compounds that may stimulate digestion and have mild analgesic effects (Krochmal et al., 1960).

However, comprehensive phytochemical analyses specific to *Lewisia rediviva* are limited. Much of the existing literature focuses on the botanical characteristics rather than detailed chemical composition.

Mechanism of Action

The potential effects of bitterroot on neuropathy are not well-documented in scientific literature. However, general mechanisms by which herbal remedies may influence neuropathic pain include:

- **Anti-inflammatory Effects**: By reducing inflammation, herbal compounds can alleviate pressure on nerves and decrease pain signals (Anand & Katz, 2010).
- **Antioxidant Properties**: Antioxidants neutralize free radicals, preventing oxidative stress that can damage nerve cells (Sas et al., 2018).

- **Modulation of Neurotransmitters**: Some plant compounds can influence neurotransmitter levels, affecting pain perception (Elsas et al., 2010).

Doses and Administration

- **Decoction**: Boiling the root to make a tea, consumed for its purported health benefits (Turner et al., 1980).
- **Poultice**: Applying crushed roots externally to affected areas (Moerman, 1998).

Due to the absence of clinical studies, no specific dosage guidelines can be recommended. Caution is advised, and consultation with a healthcare professional is essential before using bitterroot for therapeutic purposes.

History of Use

- **Nutritional Source**: The root was harvested as a valuable food resource, despite its bitter taste. It was often mixed with other foods to improve palatability (Krochmal et al., 1960).
- **Medicinal Uses**: Used traditionally to treat sore throats, toothaches, and as a general health tonic (Turner et al., 1980).
- **Cultural Significance**: Bitterroot holds spiritual importance for tribes such as the Salish, symbolizing endurance and resilience (Hart, 1976).

Evaluation of Scientific Evidence

Currently, there is a paucity of scientific studies investigating the effects of bitterroot on neuropathy. The lack of clinical trials or pharmacological research means that any claims regarding its efficacy are not supported by empirical evidence.

Conclusion

While bitterroot has historical significance and traditional uses among Native American communities, there is insufficient scientific data to substantiate its effectiveness in treating neuropathy. The bioactive compounds present in the plant suggest potential therapeutic actions, but without rigorous research, conclusions cannot be drawn. Individuals interested in exploring bitterroot for neuropathy should exercise caution and consult healthcare professionals. Future studies are necessary to elucidate the pharmacological properties and assess the safety and efficacy of bitterroot in neuropathic pain management.

BPC-157

BPC-157, also known as Body Protection Compound 157, is a synthetic peptide derived from a protein found in the human stomach. It has gained attention for its potential therapeutic benefits, particularly in tissue repair and regeneration.

Compounds Derived from BPC-157

- **BPC-157**: The primary active compound, BPC-157, is a synthetic peptide that mimics the natural peptide found in gastric juice. It is known for its regenerative and healing properties[1].

Mechanisms of Action

- **Promotion of Nerve Regeneration**: BPC-157 promotes the regeneration of nerve cells by upregulating the expression of genes involved in cell migration, differentiation, and survival. It enhances the repair of damaged nerves, which is crucial for alleviating neuropathic pain[2].
- **Anti-inflammatory Effects**: BPC-157 reduces inflammation by modulating the activity of pro-inflammatory cytokines and pathways. This helps in mitigating the inflammatory processes associated with neuropathy[3].
- **Angiogenesis and Vasculogenesis**: BPC-157 stimulates the formation of new blood vessels (angiogenesis) and the repair of existing ones (vasculogenesis). Improved blood flow to damaged nerves enhances nutrient and oxygen delivery, promoting nerve repair and reducing neuropathic pain[1].
- **Reduction of Oxidative Stress**: BPC-157 has antioxidant properties that help in reducing oxidative stress, a significant contributor to nerve damage in neuropathy[2].

Effects on Neuropathy

- **Pain Reduction**: BPC-157 has been shown to reduce neuropathic pain by promoting nerve regeneration and reducing inflammation. Studies on rodent models have demonstrated its

effectiveness in decreasing hypersensitivity and alleviating pain behaviors[3].
- **Improved Sensory Function**: By enhancing nerve repair and reducing oxidative damage, BPC-157 helps improve sensory and motor functions in individuals with neuropathy[2].
- **Prevention of Neuropathy Progression**: Regular use of BPC-157 can prevent the progression of neuropathy by maintaining adequate blood flow and reducing inflammatory and oxidative damage to nerves[1].

Dosages

The optimal dosage of BPC-157 for managing neuropathy varies, but studies suggest that doses ranging from **200 to 500 mcg per day** are generally safe and effective[3]. It is advisable to start with a lower dose and gradually increase it to monitor tolerance and effectiveness. BPC-157 is typically administered via subcutaneous or intramuscular injections. Consulting with a healthcare provider before starting supplementation is recommended to tailor the dosage to individual needs and conditions[3].

Conclusion

BPC-157, through its nerve regeneration, anti-inflammatory, and angiogenic properties, offers promising therapeutic benefits for neuropathy. Its mechanisms of action contribute to pain reduction, improved sensory function, and prevention of neuropathy progression. While more research is needed to establish optimal dosages and long-term safety, current evidence supports the potential of BPC-157 as a valuable treatment option for managing neuropathy.

Chinese Peony

Chinese peony (Paeonia lactiflora Pall.) is a perennial flowering plant native to East Asia, particularly China. It has been a cornerstone of Traditional Chinese Medicine (TCM) for over 1,500 years, used to treat various ailments due to its anti-inflammatory, analgesic, and immunomodulatory properties. Recent research has explored its potential benefits for neuropathy—a condition characterized by nerve damage resulting in pain, tingling, and numbness, often associated with diabetes and other chronic diseases.

Active Ingredients and Compounds

Chinese peony contains a variety of bioactive compounds, primarily in its roots, which contribute to its medicinal properties:

- **Paeoniflorin**: The most abundant and significant compound, comprising up to 90% of total monoterpene glycosides. It exhibits anti-inflammatory, analgesic, neuroprotective, and immunomodulatory effects.
- **Albiflorin**: Another monoterpene glycoside with similar properties to paeoniflorin, contributing to anti-inflammatory and analgesic effects.
- **Paeonol**: A phenolic compound with antioxidant, anti-inflammatory, and neuroprotective activities.
- **Flavonoids**: Such as quercetin and kaempferol, known for their antioxidant properties.
- **Tannins and Polysaccharides**: Contribute to the overall therapeutic effects by supporting immune function and providing antioxidant benefits.

Mechanism of Action

The potential benefits of Chinese peony for neuropathy are attributed to several mechanisms:

- **Anti-inflammatory Effects**: Paeoniflorin inhibits the production of pro-inflammatory cytokines (e.g., TNF-α, IL-1β, IL-6) and reduces the activation of nuclear factor-kappa B (NF-κB), a key regulator of inflammation. This reduction in inflammation can alleviate nerve damage and pain associated with neuropathy.

- **Neuroprotective Properties**: Paeoniflorin and paeonol protect neurons from oxidative stress-induced apoptosis (cell death) by enhancing antioxidant defenses and inhibiting caspase pathways involved in apoptosis.
- **Analgesic Effects**: Chinese peony compounds modulate pain perception by influencing neurotransmitter systems, such as increasing the levels of serotonin and gamma-aminobutyric acid (GABA), which have inhibitory effects on pain transmission.
- **Immunomodulation**: The herb regulates immune responses by balancing Th1/Th2 cytokine profiles, potentially reducing autoimmune-mediated nerve damage.
- **Enhancement of Blood Flow**: By improving microcirculation, Chinese peony may enhance nutrient and oxygen delivery to damaged nerves, facilitating healing.

History of Use

- **Traditional Chinese Medicine (TCM)**: Chinese peony, known as "Bai Shao," has been documented in ancient texts like the Shen Nong Ben Cao Jing (Divine Husbandman's Classic of the Materia Medica) dating back to the Han Dynasty (206 BCE–220 CE).
- **Medicinal Applications**: Traditionally used to treat pain, inflammation, menstrual disorders, and liver ailments. It is considered to nourish the blood and preserve the yin.
- **Herbal Formulations**: Often used in combination with other herbs in formulas like **Dang Gui Shao Yao San** and **Xiao Yao San** to enhance therapeutic effects.

Doses

- **Decoction (Herbal Tea)**:
    - Typical dosage: **6 to 15 grams** of dried Chinese peony root, boiled in water.
    - Usually prepared as part of a multi-herb decoction under the guidance of a TCM practitioner.
- **Powdered Extracts**:
    - Standardized extracts containing specific amounts of paeoniflorin.
    - Dosage varies; follow manufacturer's recommendations or consult a healthcare provider.
- **Capsules/Tablets**:
    - Commonly available in doses of **500 mg**.
    - Typical usage: **500 mg to 1,000 mg**, taken **2–3 times daily**.

Dosages may vary based on individua health conditions, age, and the presence of other medications. Consultation with a healthcare professional is essential for personalized dosing.

Types and How to Supplement

- **Raw Herb**:
    - **Whole Dried Root**: Used in decoctions; requires proper preparation.
    - **Sliced Root**: Easier to handle for making teas or decoctions.
- **Extracts**:
    - **Powdered Extracts**: Can be mixed with water or juice.
    - **Standardized Extracts**: Ensure consistent levels of active compounds like paeoniflorin.
- **Capsules/Tablets**:
    - Provide a convenient and precise dosing method.
    - Often used in integrative medicine practices.
- **Combination Formulas**:
    - Chinese peony is frequently included in multi-herb formulations designed to address specific health concerns.

Conclusion

Chinese peony (Paeonia lactiflora Pall.) shows promise as a natural remedy for neuropathy due to its anti-inflammatory, neuroprotective, and analgesic properties. Its rich content of bioactive compounds, particularly paeoniflorin, contributes to its therapeutic potential. While traditional use and preliminary studies are encouraging, more extensive clinical research is needed to establish definitive efficacy and safety for neuropathy treatment. Individuals interested in using Chinese peony should seek guidance from qualified healthcare professionals to ensure it aligns with their health needs and to prevent potential interactions with other medications.

Chrysanthemum

Chrysanthemum (Chrysanthemum morifolium), a flowering plant native to East Asia, has been revered for its medicinal properties in traditional Chinese medicine (TCM) for over 2,000 years. Known for its antioxidant and anti-inflammatory effects, chrysanthemum has been used to treat various ailments, including headaches, fever, and hypertension. Recently, there has been interest in its potential benefits for neuropathy, a condition characterized by nerve damage that leads to pain, tingling, and numbness.

Active Ingredients and Compounds

Chrysanthemum contains a variety of bioactive compounds that contribute to its medicinal properties:

- **Flavonoids**: Including luteolin, apigenin, and acacetin, known for their antioxidant and anti-inflammatory effects.
- **Phenolic acids**: Such as chlorogenic acid and caffeic acid, which have strong antioxidant properties.
- **Essential oils**: Containing compounds like borneol and camphor that may contribute to anti-inflammatory effects.
- **Sesquiterpene lactones**: Such as nobilin and artecanin, which may have anti-inflammatory and neuroprotective activities.
- **Vitamins and minerals**: Including vitamin A, vitamin C, potassium, and calcium.

Mechanism of Action

While direct research on chrysanthemum's effects on neuropathy is limited, its active compounds suggest potential mechanisms that may benefit nerve health:

- **Antioxidant Activity**: Flavonoids and phenolic acids in chrysanthemum help neutralize free radicals, reducing oxidative stress that can damage nerve cells. This protection may help prevent or slow the progression of neuropathy.

- **Anti-Inflammatory Effects**: The anti-inflammatory properties of chrysanthemum's compounds may reduce inflammation around nerves, potentially alleviating neuropathic pain.
- **Neuroprotective Potential**: Some studies indicate that certain flavonoids in chrysanthemum can protect neurons from damage and may promote nerve regeneration.
- **Inhibition of Nitric Oxide Production**: Excess nitric oxide can contribute to inflammation and nerve damage. Chrysanthemum extracts have been shown to inhibit nitric oxide synthesis, which may help in managing neuropathy.

History of Use

- **Traditional Chinese Medicine**: Chrysanthemum has been used to treat conditions like colds, headaches, and hypertension. It is known as a "cooling" herb that helps reduce heat and toxins in the body.
- **Eye Health**: Traditionally used to improve vision and relieve eye fatigue, which may be related to its antioxidant properties.
- **Cardiovascular Support**: Employed to lower blood pressure and improve circulation, potentially benefiting nerve health indirectly.

While not historically used explicitly for neuropathy, the general health benefits and nerve-protective properties of chrysanthemum make it a candidate for supporting nerve health.

Doses

- **Chrysanthemum Tea**:
    - Steep **1–2 teaspoons (about 2–4 grams)** of dried chrysanthemum flowers in hot water for **5–10 minutes**.
    - Consume **1–3 times daily**.
    - Can be sweetened with honey or combined with other herbs like goji berries for additional benefits.
- **Capsules/Tablets**:
    - Standard doses range from **500 mg to 1,000 mg**, taken **1–3 times daily**.
    - Follow the manufacturer's instructions or consult a healthcare provider.
- **Tinctures**:
    - Dosage can vary; typically, **10–30 drops** in water or juice, taken **2–3 times daily**.
    - Consult specific product guidelines.

Types and How to Supplement

- **Dried Flowers**: Used to make teas or infusions. Easily available in herbal shops and some grocery stores.
- **Capsules/Tablets**: Contain powdered chrysanthemum extract for convenient dosing.
- **Liquid Extracts/Tinctures**: Alcohol or glycerin-based extracts for those who prefer liquid supplements.
- **Topical Applications**: Creams or ointments containing chrysanthemum extracts may be available for external use.

Supplementation Tips:

- **Consult a Healthcare Professional**: Especially important if you are pregnant, nursing, have allergies to plants in the Asteraceae family (e.g., ragweed, daisies), or are taking other medications.
- **Choose Quality Products**: Opt for supplements from reputable manufacturers that provide third-party testing for purity and potency.
- **Start with Lower Doses**: To assess tolerance, begin with a lower dose and gradually increase as needed under professional guidance.
- **Monitor for Side Effects**: Though chrysanthemum is generally considered safe, some individuals may experience allergic reactions or gastrointestinal discomfort.

Conclusion

Chrysanthemum holds potential as a supportive herb for neuropathy due to its antioxidant, anti-inflammatory, and possible neuroprotective properties. While direct evidence is limited, the bioactive compounds in chrysanthemum may help alleviate neuropathic symptoms by protecting nerve cells and reducing inflammation. Further research is needed to establish definitive efficacy and safety. Individuals interested in using chrysanthemum for neuropathy should consult healthcare professionals to ensure it is appropriate for their specific health needs.

Coenzyme Q10

Coenzyme Q10 (CoQ10), also known as ubiquinone, is a naturally occurring antioxidant found in the mitochondria of cells. It plays a crucial role in the production of adenosine triphosphate (ATP), which is essential for cellular energy.

Compounds Derived from CoQ10

- **Ubiquinone**: The oxidized form of CoQ10, which participates in the electron transport chain within mitochondria, facilitating ATP production[1].
- **Ubiquinol**: The reduced form of CoQ10, which acts as a potent antioxidant, protecting cells from oxidative damage[2].

Mechanisms of Action

- **Mitochondrial Function**: CoQ10 is integral to the mitochondrial electron transport chain, where it helps generate ATP. This is crucial for maintaining cellular energy levels, particularly in nerve cells that have high energy demands[1].
- **Antioxidant Properties**: CoQ10, especially in its reduced form (ubiquinol), scavenges free radicals and reduces oxidative stress. This is significant in neuropathy, where oxidative damage to nerves is a common pathological feature[2].
- **Anti-inflammatory Effects**: CoQ10 can inhibit the activation of nuclear factor kappa B (NF-kB), a key player in the inflammatory response. By reducing inflammation, CoQ10 helps alleviate pain and prevent further nerve damage[3].
- **Neuroprotection**: CoQ10's ability to enhance mitochondrial function and reduce oxidative stress contributes to its neuroprotective effects. It helps in maintaining the health of neurons and preventing their degeneration[4].

Effects on Neuropathy

- **Pain Reduction**: CoQ10 supplementation has been shown to reduce neuropathic pain. This is primarily due to its antioxidant and anti-inflammatory properties, which help in mitigating the underlying causes of pain[3].

- **Improved Nerve Function**: By enhancing mitochondrial function and reducing oxidative stress, CoQ10 aids in the repair and regeneration of damaged nerves. This leads to improved sensory and motor functions in individuals with neuropathy[4].
- **Prevention of Neuropathy Progression**: Regular supplementation with CoQ10 can prevent the progression of neuropathy by maintaining adequate cellular energy levels and reducing inflammatory and oxidative damage to nerves[3].

Dosages

The optimal dosage of CoQ10 for neuropathy varies, but studies suggest that doses ranging from **100 to 300 mg per day** are generally safe and effective[5]. It is advisable to start with a lower dose and gradually increase it to monitor tolerance and effectiveness. Consulting with a healthcare provider before starting supplementation is recommended to tailor the dosage to individual needs and conditions[5].

Conclusion

Coenzyme Q10, through its roles in mitochondrial function, antioxidant defense, and anti-inflammatory action, offers promising therapeutic benefits for neuropathy. Its mechanisms of action contribute to pain reduction, improved nerve function, and prevention of neuropathy progression. While more research is needed to establish optimal dosages, current evidence supports the potential of CoQ10 as a valuable supplement in managing neuropathy.

Curcumin

Curcumin, the primary active compound in turmeric (Curcuma longa), has been extensively studied for its therapeutic properties, particularly its anti-inflammatory and antioxidant effects.

Compounds Derived from Curcumin

- **Curcuminoids**: Curcumin is part of a group of compounds known as curcuminoids, which also include demethoxycurcumin and bisdemethoxycurcumin. These compounds contribute to the overall therapeutic effects of turmeric[1].
- **Tetrahydrocurcumin**: A metabolite of curcumin, tetrahydrocurcumin, has shown potent antioxidant properties and contributes to the neuroprotective effects of curcumin[2].

Mechanisms of Action

- **Anti-inflammatory Effects**: Curcumin inhibits the activation of nuclear factor kappa B (NF-κB), a key regulator of inflammation. By suppressing NF-κB, curcumin reduces the production of pro-inflammatory cytokines such as interleukin (IL)-1β, IL-6, and tumor necrosis factor-alpha (TNF-α)[1].
- **Antioxidant Properties**: Curcumin scavenges free radicals and enhances the activity of antioxidant enzymes like superoxide dismutase (SOD) and catalase. This reduces oxidative stress, which is a significant contributor to nerve damage in neuropathy[2].
- **Neuroprotection**: Curcumin promotes the survival and growth of neurons by modulating various signaling pathways, including the mitogen-activated protein kinase (MAPK) and extracellular signal-regulated kinase (ERK) pathways[3].
- **Improved Nerve Function**: Curcumin enhances nerve regeneration and improves sensory nerve conduction velocity (SNCV), which is crucial for maintaining nerve function[3].

Effects on Neuropathy

- **Pain Reduction**: Curcumin has been shown to alleviate neuropathic pain by reducing inflammation and oxidative stress. Studies have demonstrated its effectiveness in reducing pain and improving quality of life in individuals with neuropathy[4].

- **Improved Sensory Function**: By promoting nerve regeneration and reducing oxidative damage, curcumin helps improve sensory and motor functions in individuals with neuropathy[3].
- **Prevention of Neuropathy Progression**: Regular supplementation with curcumin can prevent the progression of neuropathy by maintaining adequate antioxidant defenses and reducing inflammatory damage to nerves[4].

Dosages

The optimal dosage of curcumin for neuropathy varies, but studies suggest that doses ranging from **500 to 2000 mg per day** are generally safe and effective. It is advisable to start with a lower dose and gradually increase it to monitor tolerance and effectiveness. Curcumin is often taken with black pepper extract (piperine) to enhance its bioavailability. Consulting with a healthcare provider before starting supplementation is recommended to tailor the dosage to individual needs and conditions.

Conclusion

Curcumin, through its anti-inflammatory, antioxidant, and neuroprotective properties, offers promising therapeutic benefits for neuropathy. Its mechanisms of action contribute to pain reduction, improved nerve function, and prevention of neuropathy progression. While more research is needed to establish optimal dosages, current evidence supports the potential of curcumin as a valuable supplement in managing neuropathy.

Dandelion

Taraxacum officinale, commonly known as **dandelion**, has been used in traditional medicine for centuries. Dandelion is a common weed that grows in everyone's yard. This is one of the best supplements hidden in plain sight.

Compounds and Ingredients

Dandelion is rich in bioactive compounds that may contribute to its medicinal properties:

- **Vitamins and Minerals**: High levels of vitamin A, vitamin C, vitamin K, several B vitamins, and minerals such as iron, calcium, magnesium, and potassium (Schütz et al., 2006).
- **Phytochemicals**:
    - **Sesquiterpene Lactones**: Including taraxinic acid and taraxasterol, known for anti-inflammatory properties (Martinez et al., 2015).
    - **Flavonoids**: Such as luteolin and apigenin, which possess antioxidant effects (Hu & Kitts, 2005).
    - **Phenolic Acids:** Including chicoric acid and chlorogenic acid, contributing to antioxidant activity (Schütz et al., 2006).
    - **Polysaccharides**: Inulin, a prebiotic fiber that supports gut health and may influence immune function (Martinez et al., 2015).

Mechanism of Action

While specific studies on dandelion's effects on neuropathy are limited, its bioactive compounds suggest potential mechanisms that could alleviate neuropathic symptoms:

- **Anti-inflammatory Effects**: Dandelion's sesquiterpene lactones and flavonoids may reduce inflammation by inhibiting pro-inflammatory cytokines and enzymes like COX-2, involved in pain signaling (Schütz et al., 2006).
- **Antioxidant Activity**: Flavonoids and phenolic acids scavenge free radicals, reducing oxidative stress that can damage nerve cells (Hu & Kitts, 2005).
- **Neuroprotective Properties**: Antioxidants may protect neurons from degeneration, potentially slowing the progression of neuropathy.
- **Improving Microcirculation**: Dandelion may enhance blood flow, providing better oxygen and nutrient delivery to affected nerves (Blumenthal et al., 2000).
- **Immune Modulation**: Certain compounds may modulate immune responses, decreasing autoimmune reactions that contribute to nerve inflammation.

Potential Effects on Neuropathy

Though direct clinical evidence is scarce, the combined anti-inflammatory and antioxidant properties of dandelion could theoretically help in managing neuropathic pain and promoting nerve health:

- **Pain Reduction:** By decreasing inflammation and oxidative stress, dandelion may alleviate pain associated with neuropathy.
- **Nerve Repair**: Enhanced antioxidant defenses may support the repair and regeneration of damaged nerve tissues.
- **Symptom Relief**: Improved circulation and reduced inflammation could lessen symptoms like tingling and numbness.

Doses and Administration

There is no standardized dosage of dandelion for neuropathy, and recommendations vary based on the form used:

- **Tea**: Steep 1-2 teaspoons of dried dandelion root or leaves in hot water for 5-10 minutes, consumed 2-3 times daily.
- **Tincture**: 2-5 ml of dandelion tincture (1:5 ratio in 45% alcohol) taken 2-3 times daily.
- **Capsules/Tablets**: Standardized extracts, often 500 mg per capsule, with a common dose of 500-1,000 mg taken 1-3 times daily.
- **Fresh Leaves**: Consumed in salads or cooked as greens.

Safety and Precautions

- **Allergies**: Individuals allergic to plants in the Asteraceae family (e.g., ragweed, chrysanthemums, marigolds) may experience allergic reactions (Brinker, 2010).
- **Drug Interactions**: Dandelion may interact with medications, including diuretics, antibiotics, and blood sugar medications. Consultation with a healthcare provider is essential (Brinker, 2010).
- **Pregnancy and Lactation**: Safety has not been established; use cautiously and under professional guidance.

History of Use

- **Traditional Medicine**: Dandelion has been used in traditional Chinese medicine, Native American medicine, and European herbal practices.
- **Medicinal Uses**:
    - *Diuretic*: Known as "pissenlit" in French, reflecting its diuretic properties (Clare et al., 2009).
    - *Digestive Aid*: Used to stimulate appetite and aid digestion.
    - *Liver and Gallbladder Support*: Employed to promote liver detoxification and bile production.
- Cultural Significance: Considered both a nutritional food source and a medicinal herb for centuries.

Conclusion

Dandelion's rich composition of anti-inflammatory and antioxidant compounds presents a plausible basis for its potential benefits in managing neuropathy. While traditional use and theoretical mechanisms are encouraging, clinical studies specifically investigating dandelion's efficacy for neuropathy are lacking. Therefore, it should be used cautiously, and individuals should consult healthcare professionals before incorporating dandelion into their treatment regimen. Further research is necessary to substantiate its effectiveness and establish appropriate dosing guidelines.

GABA

Gamma-aminobutyric acid (GABA) is the primary inhibitory neurotransmitter in the central nervous system (CNS). It plays a crucial role in maintaining the balance between excitatory and inhibitory signals in the brain.

What is GABA?

GABA is a naturally occurring amino acid that functions as a neurotransmitter in the brain. It is responsible for reducing neuronal excitability throughout the nervous system. GABA is synthesized from glutamate through the action of the enzyme glutamate decarboxylase[1].

Effects on Neuropathy

Neuropathy, particularly peripheral neuropathy, involves damage to the peripheral nerves, leading to symptoms such as pain, tingling, and numbness. GABA has shown potential in managing neuropathic pain through several mechanisms:

- **Pain Modulation**: GABAergic neurons play a critical role in modulating pain signals within the spinal cord and brain. By enhancing GABAergic signaling, it is possible to inhibit the activation of pain-signaling neurons, thereby reducing pain perception[2].
- **Neuroprotection**: GABA has neuroprotective properties that help protect neurons from damage caused by oxidative stress and inflammation. This is particularly important in neuropathy, where nerve damage is a key issue[2].
- **Reduction of Hyperexcitability**: Neuropathic pain often involves hyperexcitability of neurons. GABA helps to reduce this hyperexcitability by increasing inhibitory signals, which can help alleviate pain and discomfort associated with neuropathy[2].

Active Compounds and Mechanisms of Action

The beneficial effects of GABA on neuropathy are primarily attributed to its role as an inhibitory neurotransmitter. Here's how GABA and its related compounds work:

- **GABA Receptors**: GABA exerts its effects by binding to GABA receptors, specifically GABA_A and GABA_B receptors. Activation of these receptors leads to the opening of ion channels that allow chloride ions to enter the neuron, making it more negatively charged and less likely to fire an action potential[3].
- **Gabapentin and Pregabalin**: These are GABA analogs that are commonly used to treat neuropathic pain. They do not directly activate GABA receptors but instead bind to the α2δ subunit of voltage-gated calcium channels in the CNS. This binding reduces the release of excitatory neurotransmitters, thereby reducing neuronal excitability and pain[4].
- **Antioxidant Properties**: GABA and its analogs have been shown to have antioxidant properties, which help protect neurons from oxidative stress. This is particularly beneficial in neuropathy, where oxidative damage can exacerbate nerve injury[2].
- **Anti-Inflammatory Effects**: GABAergic signaling can also reduce inflammation, which is a common contributor to neuropathic pain. By reducing inflammatory responses, GABA helps to protect nerves from further damage[2].

Conclusion

GABA plays a significant role in managing neuropathic pain through its inhibitory effects on neuronal excitability, neuroprotective properties, and ability to reduce inflammation and oxidative stress. GABA and its analogs, such as gabapentin and pregabalin, offer promising therapeutic options for individuals suffering from neuropathy. However, it is important to use these treatments under the guidance of a healthcare professional to ensure safety and efficacy.

Sources

Gamma-Linolenic Acid (GLA)

Gamma-Linolenic Acid (GLA) is an **omega-6 fatty acid** found in various plant oils, such as evening primrose oil, borage oil, and blackcurrant seed oil. It has garnered attention for its potential therapeutic effects on neuropathy, particularly diabetic neuropathy.

Compounds Derived from GLA

- **Dihomo-Gamma-Linolenic Acid (DGLA)**: Once absorbed, GLA is converted into DGLA, which serves as a precursor to several anti-inflammatory lipid mediators[1].
- **Prostaglandin E1 (PGE1)**: DGLA is further metabolized into PGE1, a potent anti-inflammatory compound that helps reduce inflammation and improve blood flow[1].

Mechanisms of Action

- **Anti-inflammatory Effects**: GLA and its metabolites, such as PGE1, exhibit strong anti-inflammatory properties. They inhibit the production of pro-inflammatory cytokines and reduce inflammation, which is a key factor in the progression of neuropathy[1].
- **Improved Nerve Blood Flow**: GLA enhances the production of PGE1, which acts as a vasodilator, improving blood flow to peripheral nerves. This increased blood flow helps deliver essential nutrients and oxygen, aiding in nerve repair and function[2].
- **Neuroprotection**: GLA's anti-inflammatory and antioxidant properties contribute to its neuroprotective effects. By reducing oxidative stress and inflammation, GLA helps protect nerves from damage and supports their regeneration[2].
- **Modulation of Lipid Metabolism**: GLA influences lipid metabolism, leading to the production of anti-inflammatory lipid mediators that help in maintaining nerve health and function[1].

Effects on Neuropathy

- **Pain Reduction**: GLA supplementation has been shown to reduce pain associated with neuropathy. This is primarily due to its anti-

inflammatory effects and the subsequent improvement in nerve function[2].
- **Improved Nerve Function**: By enhancing blood flow and reducing oxidative stress, GLA aids in the repair and regeneration of damaged nerves. This leads to improved sensory and motor functions in individuals with neuropathy[2].
- **Prevention of Neuropathy Progression**: Regular supplementation with GLA can prevent the progression of neuropathy by maintaining adequate blood flow and reducing inflammatory and oxidative damage to nerves[2].

Dosages

The optimal dosage of GLA for neuropathy varies, but studies suggest that doses ranging from **300 to 600 mg per day** are generally safe and effective[2]. It is advisable to start with a lower dose and gradually increase it to monitor tolerance and effectiveness. Consulting with a healthcare provider before starting supplementation is recommended to tailor the dosage to individual needs and conditions[2].

Conclusion

Gamma-Linolenic Acid (GLA), through its conversion to DGLA and subsequent production of anti-inflammatory mediators like PGE1, offers promising therapeutic benefits for neuropathy. Its mechanisms of action, including anti-inflammatory effects, improved nerve blood flow, and neuroprotection, contribute to pain reduction, improved nerve function, and prevention of neuropathy progression. While more research is needed to establish optimal dosages, current evidence supports the potential of GLA as a valuable supplement in managing neuropathy.

Ginkgo Biloba

Ginkgo biloba, one of the oldest living tree species, has been used for centuries in traditional Chinese medicine. Extracts from its leaves are popular supplements known for their potential to enhance cognitive function and improve circulation. Recent research has explored Ginkgo biloba's effects on neuropathy—a condition characterized by nerve damage that leads to pain, tingling, and numbness, often in the hands and feet.

Active Ingredients and Compounds

The primary active components of Ginkgo biloba extract (GBE) include:

- **Flavonoids**: Such as quercetin, kaempferol, and isorhamnetin. These are potent antioxidants that protect nerve cells from oxidative damage.
- **Terpene Lactones**: Including ginkgolides (A, B, C, J) and bilobalide. These compounds are unique to Ginkgo biloba and contribute to its neuroprotective and anti-inflammatory effects.

Mechanism of Action

Ginkgo biloba's potential benefits for neuropathy stem from several mechanisms:

- **Antioxidant Effects**: Flavonoids in GBE scavenge free radicals, reducing oxidative stress that can damage peripheral nerves.
- **Neuroprotective Properties**: Ginkgolides and bilobalide protect neurons by inhibiting apoptosis (programmed cell death) and promoting nerve regeneration.
- **Anti-inflammatory Action**: GBE reduces the production of pro-inflammatory cytokines, which may help alleviate neuropathic pain.
- **Improved Microcirculation**: GBE enhances blood flow by dilating blood vessels and reducing blood viscosity, improving oxygen and nutrient delivery to nerves.
- **Modulation of Neurotransmitters**: GBE may influence neurotransmitter systems, including serotonin and GABA, which play roles in pain perception and nerve function.

History of Use

Ginkgo biloba has been used in traditional Chinese medicine for over 2,000 years. Historically, it was utilized to treat ailments such as cognitive decline, respiratory issues, and circulatory disorders. In modern times, GBE has gained popularity worldwide as a natural supplement for enhancing memory, cognitive function, and peripheral circulation.

Doses

For neuropathy, a common recommended dosage of standardized Ginkgo biloba extract is **120 to 240 mg per day**, divided into two or three doses. The extract should be standardized to contain **24% flavone glycosides** and **6% terpene lactones** to ensure consistent potency and efficacy.

Types and How to Supplement

- **Standardized Capsules/Tablets**: Contain measured amounts of active ingredients for consistent dosing.
- **Liquid Extracts/Tinctures**: Offer flexibility in dosing but require careful measurement.
- **Teas**: Made from Ginkgo leaves but may have lower concentrations of active compounds.

Conclusion

Ginkgo biloba shows promise as a natural supplement for managing neuropathy due to its antioxidant, neuroprotective, anti-inflammatory, and circulatory benefits. While preliminary studies are encouraging, more extensive clinical trials are needed to establish definitive efficacy and safety. Individuals considering Ginkgo biloba supplementation should consult healthcare professionals to ensure it aligns with their health needs and to avoid potential interactions with medications.

Hawthorn

Hawthorn (Crataegus spp.) is a flowering shrub or small tree belonging to the Rosaceae family. It has been used for centuries in traditional medicine, particularly for cardiovascular health. Known for its antioxidant, anti-inflammatory, and vasodilatory properties, hawthorn has attracted interest for its potential benefits in various health conditions. Recent research suggests that hawthorn may also have positive effects on neuropathy—a condition characterized by nerve damage that leads to pain, tingling, and numbness, often associated with diabetes and other chronic diseases.

Active Ingredients and Compounds

Hawthorn contains a variety of bioactive compounds that contribute to its medicinal properties:

- **Flavonoids**: Such as quercetin, hyperoside, vitexin, rutin, and epicatechin. These potent antioxidants help protect nerve cells from oxidative stress and may improve blood circulation.
- **Oligomeric Proanthocyanidins (OPCs)**: Powerful antioxidants that support vascular health by strengthening blood vessel walls and improving capillary permeability.
- **Triterpenic Acids**: Including ursolic acid and oleanolic acid, which have anti-inflammatory and analgesic properties.
- **Phenolic Acids**: Such as chlorogenic acid and caffeic acid, contributing to antioxidant effects.

Mechanism of Action

Hawthorn's potential benefits for neuropathy are attributed to several mechanisms:

- **Antioxidant Effects**: Hawthorn's flavonoids and OPCs scavenge free radicals, reducing oxidative stress that can damage nerve cells. Oxidative stress is a key factor in the development and progression of neuropathy.

- **Anti-inflammatory Properties**: By inhibiting the production of pro-inflammatory cytokines, hawthorn may reduce inflammation in nerve tissues, alleviating neuropathic pain.
- **Improved Circulation**: Hawthorn enhances blood flow by dilating blood vessels and decreasing vascular resistance. Improved microcirculation can lead to better oxygen and nutrient delivery to damaged nerves, promoting healing and regeneration.
- **Neuroprotective Effects**: Some studies suggest that hawthorn's compounds may protect neurons from injury and support nerve regeneration by modulating signaling pathways involved in cell survival.

History of Use

- **Traditional Medicine**: Hawthorn has been used in traditional Chinese medicine (TCM) and European herbal medicine for centuries. In TCM, known as "Shan Zha," it is used to aid digestion and improve cardiovascular health.
- **Cardiovascular Use**: Historically, hawthorn has been primarily used for heart-related conditions, such as heart failure, hypertension, and arrhythmias, due to its positive inotropic and vasodilatory effects.
- **Extension to Neuropathy**: While not traditionally used specifically for neuropathy, the recognition of hawthorn's antioxidant and anti-inflammatory properties has led to interest in its potential application for neuropathic conditions.

Doses

- **Standardized Extracts**: Common dosages range from **160 to 900 mg per day**, divided into two or three doses. Extracts should be standardized to contain **2–3% flavonoids** or **18–20% OPCs** to ensure consistency and efficacy.
- **Herbal Tea**: Hawthorn can be consumed as a tea by steeping **1–2 teaspoons (4–5 grams)** of dried berries, leaves, or flowers in boiling water for 10–15 minutes, consumed up to three times daily.
- **Capsules/Tablets**: Follow the manufacturer's recommended dosage, typically **300–600 mg** taken two to three times daily.

It's essential to consult a healthcare professional before starting hawthorn supplementation, especially for individuals taking medications or managing chronic conditions.

Types and How to Supplement

Capsules/Tablets: Contain powdered hawthorn berries, leaves, or flowers for convenient dosing. **Standardized Extracts**: Provide consistent levels of active compounds. **Tinctures**: Alcohol-based extracts that may offer quicker absorption. **Teas**: Made from dried hawthorn parts for a milder effect.

Conclusion

Hawthorn's rich composition of antioxidants and bioactive compounds positions it as a promising supplement for supporting nerve health and potentially managing neuropathy. Its antioxidant, anti-inflammatory, and circulatory benefits may help alleviate neuropathic symptoms by protecting nerve cells, reducing inflammation, and improving blood flow. While preliminary studies and traditional use suggest potential benefits, more comprehensive clinical research is needed to establish definitive efficacy and safety for neuropathy treatment. Individuals considering hawthorn supplementation should consult healthcare professionals to ensure it aligns with their health needs and to prevent potential interactions with medications.

L-Arginine

L-Arginine, a semi-essential amino acid, plays a crucial role in various physiological processes, including protein synthesis, immune function, and the production of nitric oxide (NO). Its potential therapeutic effects on neuropathy, particularly diabetic neuropathy, have garnered significant interest in recent years.

Compounds Derived from L-Arginine

- **Nitric Oxide (NO)**: L-Arginine is a precursor to nitric oxide, a potent vasodilator that enhances blood flow and oxygen delivery to tissues. This property is particularly beneficial in neuropathy, where improved blood flow can aid in nerve repair and function[1].
- **Agmatine**: A metabolite of L-Arginine, agmatine has shown neuroprotective properties. It modulates several key pathways involved in neuropathy, including the inhibition of NMDA receptors and the activation of the Nrf2 pathway[2].
- **Polyamines**: These are organic compounds derived from L-Arginine that play a role in cell growth and differentiation. They have been implicated in neuroprotection and the modulation of ion channels[3].

Mechanisms of Action

- **Vasodilation and Improved Blood Flow**: The primary mechanism by which L-Arginine exerts its effects on neuropathy is through the production of nitric oxide. NO-induced vasodilation improves blood flow to peripheral nerves, enhancing oxygen and nutrient delivery, which is crucial for nerve repair and function[1].
- **Neuroprotection**: Agmatine, derived from L-Arginine, offers neuroprotective benefits by reducing oxidative stress and inflammation. It inhibits the NMDA receptors, which are involved in excitotoxicity, a process that can lead to nerve damage[2].
- **Anti-inflammatory Effects**: L-Arginine and its metabolites can reduce inflammation, a key factor in the progression of neuropathy. By modulating inflammatory pathways, these compounds help in alleviating pain and preventing further nerve damage[2].
- **Antioxidant Properties**: L-Arginine and its derivatives enhance the body's antioxidant defenses, reducing oxidative stress, which is a significant contributor to nerve damage in neuropathy[2].

Effects on Neuropathy

- **Pain Reduction**: L-Arginine supplementation has been shown to reduce pain associated with neuropathy. This is primarily due to its vasodilatory effects and the subsequent improvement in nerve function[4].
- **Improved Nerve Function**: By enhancing blood flow and reducing oxidative stress, L-Arginine helps in the repair and regeneration of damaged nerves. This leads to improved sensory and motor functions in individuals with neuropathy[1].
- **Prevention of Neuropathy Progression**: Regular supplementation with L-Arginine can prevent the progression of neuropathy by maintaining adequate blood flow and reducing inflammatory and oxidative damage to nerves[4].

Conclusion

L-Arginine and its derivatives, such as nitric oxide and agmatine, offer promising therapeutic benefits for neuropathy. Through mechanisms involving vasodilation, neuroprotection, anti-inflammatory effects, and antioxidant properties, L-Arginine helps in reducing pain, improving nerve function, and preventing the progression of neuropathy. Further research is warranted to fully elucidate these mechanisms and translate these findings into clinical practice, offering hope for individuals suffering from neuropathy.

L-Citrulline

L-Citrulline, a non-essential amino acid, is gaining attention for its potential therapeutic effects on neuropathy. This is a supplement that I add to my daily stack. I use this in my preworkout for a better pump in the gym. Citrulline is one of the best N.O. producers.

Compounds Derived from L-Citrulline

- **L-Arginine**: L-Citrulline is converted into L-Arginine in the kidneys. L-Arginine is a precursor to nitric oxide (NO), a molecule that plays a crucial role in vascular health by promoting vasodilation and improving blood flow[1].
- **Nitric Oxide (NO)**: As a result of L-Arginine conversion, nitric oxide is produced. NO is essential for maintaining vascular tone and health, which is particularly beneficial in conditions like neuropathy where blood flow to nerves is compromised[2].

Mechanisms of Action

- **Vasodilation and Improved Blood Flow**: The primary mechanism by which L-Citrulline exerts its effects is through the production of nitric oxide. NO-induced vasodilation enhances blood flow, which is crucial for delivering oxygen and nutrients to peripheral nerves, aiding in their repair and function[2].
- **Reduction of Oxidative Stress**: L-Citrulline has antioxidant properties that help reduce oxidative stress, a significant contributor to nerve damage in neuropathy. By scavenging free radicals, L-Citrulline helps protect nerves from oxidative damage[3].
- **Anti-inflammatory Effects**: L-Citrulline can modulate inflammatory pathways, reducing inflammation that exacerbates neuropathy. This anti-inflammatory action helps in alleviating pain and preventing further nerve damage[4].
- **Enhancement of Nitric Oxide Production**: By increasing the availability of L-Arginine, L-Citrulline indirectly boosts nitric oxide production, which is vital for maintaining healthy blood vessels and nerve function[1].

Effects on Neuropathy

- **Pain Reduction**: L-Citrulline supplementation has been shown to reduce pain associated with neuropathy. This is primarily due to its vasodilatory effects and the subsequent improvement in nerve function[2].
- **Improved Nerve Function**: Enhanced blood flow and reduced oxidative stress contribute to the repair and regeneration of damaged nerves, leading to improved sensory and motor functions in individuals with neuropathy[3].
- **Prevention of Neuropathy Progression**: Regular supplementation with L-Citrulline can prevent the progression of neuropathy by maintaining adequate blood flow and reducing inflammatory and oxidative damage to nerves[4].

Dosages

The optimal dosage of L-Citrulline for neuropathy is not well-established, but studies suggest that doses ranging from **3 to 6 grams per day** are generally safe and effective[5]. It is advisable to start with a lower dose and gradually increase it to monitor tolerance and effectiveness. Consulting with a healthcare provider before starting supplementation is recommended to tailor the dosage to individual needs and conditions[5].

Conclusion

L-Citrulline, through its conversion to L-Arginine and subsequent production of nitric oxide, offers promising therapeutic benefits for neuropathy. Its mechanisms of action, including vasodilation, reduction of oxidative stress, and anti-inflammatory effects, contribute to pain reduction, improved nerve function, and prevention of neuropathy progression. While more research is needed to establish optimal dosages, current evidence supports the potential of L-Citrulline as a valuable supplement in managing neuropathy.

Lion's Mane

Lion's Mane (Hericium erinaceus) is a medicinal mushroom known for its neuroprotective and neuroregenerative properties. Lions's mane is a very good supplement for the brain, see my book "maximize your brain power" for more info directly relating to brain health.

Compounds Derived from Lion's Mane

- **Hericenones**: These compounds are found in the fruiting body of Lion's Mane and are known to stimulate the production of nerve growth factor (NGF), which is essential for the growth and maintenance of neurons[1].
- **Erinacines**: Found in the mycelium of Lion's Mane, erinacines are potent stimulators of NGF synthesis. They play a crucial role in promoting nerve regeneration and repair[2].
- **Polysaccharides**: These bioactive compounds have antioxidant properties that protect neurons from oxidative stress and inflammation[3].

Mechanisms of Action

- **Neurogenesis and Neuroprotection**: Lion's Mane stimulates the production of NGF, which supports the growth, maintenance, and survival of neurons. This is particularly beneficial in neuropathy, where nerve damage and degeneration are prevalent[1].
- **Anti-inflammatory Effects**: The polysaccharides and other bioactive compounds in Lion's Mane reduce inflammation by inhibiting the production of pro-inflammatory cytokines. This helps alleviate pain and prevent further nerve damage[3].
- **Antioxidant Properties**: Lion's Mane has strong antioxidant effects that protect nerve cells from oxidative stress, a significant contributor to neuropathy. By scavenging free radicals, it helps maintain neuronal health[3].
- **Enhanced Nerve Regeneration**: The hericenones and erinacines in Lion's Mane promote the regeneration of damaged nerves, improving sensory and motor functions[2].

Effects on Neuropathy

- **Pain Reduction**: Lion's Mane supplementation has been shown to reduce neuropathic pain by decreasing inflammation and oxidative stress. Studies have demonstrated its effectiveness in alleviating pain and improving quality of life in individuals with neuropathy[4].
- **Improved Sensory Function**: By promoting nerve regeneration and reducing oxidative damage, Lion's Mane helps improve sensory and motor functions in individuals with neuropathy[2].
- **Prevention of Neuropathy Progression**: Regular supplementation with Lion's Mane can prevent the progression of neuropathy by maintaining adequate levels of NGF and reducing inflammatory and oxidative damage to nerves[1].

Dosages

The optimal dosage of Lion's Mane for neuropathy varies, but studies suggest that doses ranging from **500 to 3000 mg per day** are generally safe and effective[4]. It is advisable to start with a lower dose and gradually increase it to monitor tolerance and effectiveness. Consulting with a healthcare provider before starting supplementation is recommended to tailor the dosage to individual needs and conditions[4].

Conclusion

Lion's Mane, through its neuroprotective, anti-inflammatory, and antioxidant properties, offers promising therapeutic benefits for neuropathy. Its mechanisms of action contribute to pain reduction, improved nerve function, and prevention of neuropathy progression. While more research is needed to establish optimal dosages, current evidence supports the potential of Lion's Mane as a valuable supplement in managing neuropathy.

Magnesium

Magnesium, an essential mineral involved in numerous physiological processes, has garnered attention for its potential role in alleviating neuropathic symptoms. Magnesium (Mg) is the fourth most abundant mineral in the human body and is involved in over 300 enzymatic reactions (Gröber et al., 2015).

It plays a crucial role in:

- **Energy Production**: Involved in ATP synthesis.

- **Protein Synthesis**: Essential for the formation of proteins from amino acids.

- **Nerve Function**: Regulates neurotransmitter release and neuromuscular conduction.

- **Muscle Function**: Facilitates muscle contraction and relaxation.

- **Structural Development**: Contributes to bone health and DNA/RNA synthesis.

Different Types of Magnesium Supplements

Various forms of magnesium supplements are available, differing in bioavailability and specific uses:

- **Magnesium Oxide**: Contains a high percentage of elemental magnesium but has lower absorption rates (Walker et al., 2003).

- **Magnesium Citrate**: Highly bioavailable, commonly used for magnesium deficiency (Song et al., 2012).

- **Magnesium Glycinate**: Known for better absorption and less likelihood of causing diarrhea; beneficial for neurological conditions (Schuette et al., 1994).

- **Magnesium L-Threonate**: Crosses the blood-brain barrier more effectively, potentially enhancing cognitive function (Slutsky et al., 2010).

- **Magnesium Malate**: May help with muscle pain and fatigue (Abraham & Flechas, 1992).

- **Magnesium Chloride**: Well-absorbed, used for both oral and topical applications.

Mechanism of Action

Magnesium's potential effects on neuropathy are attributed to several mechanisms:

- **NMDA Receptor Antagonism**: Magnesium blocks N-methyl-D-aspartate (NMDA) receptors, which, when overactivated, contribute to neuropathic pain through excitotoxicity (Weglicki et al., 1992).

- **Anti-inflammatory Effects**: Magnesium deficiency is associated with increased production of pro-inflammatory cytokines (e.g., TNF-α, IL-1β) (Nielsen, 2010). Adequate magnesium may reduce inflammation that exacerbates neuropathic pain.

- **Calcium Channel Regulation**: Magnesium competes with calcium ions, helping to regulate calcium influx into neurons, which can reduce neuronal hyperexcitability (Iseri & French, 1984).

- **Oxidative Stress Reduction**: Magnesium has antioxidant properties that help mitigate oxidative stress, which contributes to nerve damage (Barbosa et al., 2012).

- **Improvement of Endothelial Function**: Enhances blood flow and oxygen delivery to nerves, potentially supporting nerve repair (Maier et al., 2004).

Effects on Neuropathy

Research suggests that magnesium supplementation may alleviate neuropathic symptoms:

- **Pain Reduction**: Studies indicate that magnesium can decrease pain intensity in neuropathic conditions by modulating NMDA receptors and reducing inflammation (Freguin-Bouilland et al., 2013).

- **Nerve Protection**: Magnesium's antioxidant effects may protect nerve cells from damage and support regeneration (Bahgat et al., 2016).

- **Improved Nerve Conduction**: Adequate magnesium levels are essential for proper nerve signal transmission (Caddell, 1996).

Doses

The Recommended Dietary Allowance (RDA) for magnesium varies by age and sex:

- Adult Men (19-30 years): 400 mg/day

- Adult Women (19-30 years): 310 mg/day

- Adult Men (31+ years): 420 mg/day

- Adult Women (31+ years): 320 mg/day

(Source: National Institutes of Health [NIH], Office of Dietary Supplements, 2021)

For therapeutic uses in neuropathy, studies have used varying doses:

- **Magnesium Citrate/Glycinate**: 200-400 mg taken orally once or twice daily.

- **Magnesium L-Threonate**: Dose varies; typically, around 1,000-2,000 mg per day, divided into multiple doses.

Note: Excessive magnesium supplementation (>350 mg/day from supplements) can lead to side effects such as diarrhea, nausea, and abdominal cramping. Dosing should be individualized and supervised by a healthcare professional.

Which Type is Best for Neuropathy

- **Magnesium Glycinate**: Preferred for neurological conditions due to high bioavailability and minimal laxative effects (Schuette et al., 1994).

- **Magnesium L-Threonate**: Notable for its ability to cross the blood-brain barrier, potentially offering benefits for central sensitization in neuropathic pain (Slutsky et al., 2010).

- **Magnesium Malate**: May be beneficial if muscle pain and fatigue are prominent symptoms (Abraham & Flechas, 1992).

History of Use

Magnesium has been used medicinally since ancient times:

- **Early Use**: Epsom salts (magnesium sulfate) were used in the 17th century for their laxative properties.

- **20th Century**: Recognition of magnesium's role in neuromuscular function led to its use in treating eclampsia and cardiac arrhythmias (Altura & Altura, 1984).

- **Recent Applications**: Interest has grown in using magnesium for neurological disorders, including migraine, depression, and neuropathic pain.

Conclusion

Magnesium plays a vital role in numerous physiological processes, including nerve function. Its potential benefits for neuropathy are supported by mechanisms involving NMDA receptor antagonism, anti-inflammatory effects, calcium regulation, and antioxidant properties. Magnesium glycinate and magnesium L-Threonate are considered optimal for neurological conditions due to their high bioavailability and effectiveness. While promising, magnesium supplementation should be approached cautiously, with attention to appropriate dosing and under the guidance of a healthcare professional. Further research is warranted to establish standardized treatment protocols.

N-Acetyl cysteine (NAC)

N-Acetylcysteine (NAC) is a powerful antioxidant and precursor to glutathione, widely recognized for its therapeutic potential in various neurological disorders, including neuropathy.

What is N-Acetylcysteine (NAC)?

NAC is a modified form of the amino acid cysteine. It is commonly used as a supplement to boost antioxidant levels in the body and is also known for its role in treating acetaminophen overdose[1]. NAC is both water- and fat-soluble, allowing it to cross cell membranes and exert its effects throughout the body[1].

Effects on Neuropathy

Neuropathy, particularly peripheral neuropathy, involves damage to the peripheral nerves, leading to symptoms such as pain, tingling, and numbness. NAC has shown promise in alleviating these symptoms through several mechanisms:

- **Pain Reduction**: Clinical studies have demonstrated that NAC can significantly reduce neuropathic pain. It helps alleviate symptoms by reducing oxidative stress and inflammation, which are key contributors to nerve damage[2].
- **Improved Nerve Function**: NAC has been shown to improve nerve conduction and function. This is particularly beneficial for individuals with diabetic neuropathy, as it helps restore normal nerve activity[2].
- **Neuroprotection**: NAC provides neuroprotective effects by safeguarding nerve cells from further damage. This is achieved through its antioxidant properties, which help reduce oxidative stress and inflammation[2].

Active Compounds and Mechanisms of Action

The beneficial effects of NAC on neuropathy are primarily attributed to its role in cellular metabolism and its neuroprotective properties.

Here's how NAC and its related compounds work:

- **Glutathione Precursor**: NAC is a precursor to glutathione, one of the most important antioxidants in the body. Glutathione helps neutralize free radicals and reduce oxidative stress, protecting nerve cells from damage[3]. By boosting glutathione levels, NAC enhances the body's overall antioxidant defense system.
- **Antioxidant Properties**: NAC acts as a powerful antioxidant, neutralizing free radicals that cause oxidative stress. This helps protect nerve cells from damage and supports their repair[3].
- **Anti-Inflammatory Effects**: NAC reduces inflammation by inhibiting the activation of nuclear factor-kappa B (NF-κB), a protein complex that plays a key role in regulating the immune response to inflammation[3]. By reducing inflammation, NAC helps alleviate pain and prevent further nerve damage.
- **Regulation of Glutamate**: NAC modulates glutamate levels in the brain. Glutamate is an excitatory neurotransmitter that, in excess, can cause excitotoxicity and nerve damage. By regulating glutamate levels, NAC helps protect neurons from excitotoxicity[4].
- **Improved Blood Flow**: NAC improves microcirculation, which is crucial for delivering nutrients and oxygen to nerve cells. Enhanced blood flow helps support nerve health and function[4].

Conclusion

N-Acetylcysteine (NAC) is a versatile compound with significant potential benefits for managing neuropathy. Its role as a glutathione precursor, antioxidant, and anti-inflammatory agent, along with its ability to regulate glutamate levels and improve blood flow, makes it a valuable supplement for individuals suffering from neuropathic pain. However, it is important to use NAC under the guidance of a healthcare professional to ensure safety and efficacy.

Omega-3 Fatty Acids

Omega-3 fatty acids, primarily found in fish oil, flaxseed, and walnuts, are essential polyunsaturated fats known for their anti-inflammatory and neuroprotective properties.

Compounds Derived from Omega-3 Fatty Acids

- **Eicosapentaenoic Acid (EPA)**: EPA is known for its anti-inflammatory effects and plays a crucial role in reducing inflammation, which is beneficial in managing neuropathy[1].
- **Docosahexaenoic Acid (DHA)**: DHA is a major structural component of neuronal membranes and is essential for maintaining neuronal function and integrity[2].
- **Alpha-Linolenic Acid (ALA)**: ALA is a plant-based omega-3 fatty acid that can be converted into EPA and DHA in the body, though the conversion rate is relatively low[3].

Mechanisms of Action

- **Anti-inflammatory Effects**: Omega-3 fatty acids reduce the production of pro-inflammatory cytokines and eicosanoids. EPA and DHA inhibit the activity of enzymes like cyclooxygenase (COX) and lipoxygenase (LOX), which are involved in the inflammatory process[1].
- **Neuroprotection**: DHA is crucial for the maintenance of neuronal membranes and promotes the survival and growth of neurons. It also helps in the formation of neuroprotectin D1, a compound that protects neurons from oxidative stress and inflammation[2].
- **Improved Nerve Function**: Omega-3 fatty acids enhance nerve conduction velocity and support the regeneration of damaged nerves. They also improve the fluidity of neuronal membranes, which is essential for proper nerve signaling[4].
- **Reduction of Oxidative Stress**: Omega-3 fatty acids have antioxidant properties that help reduce oxidative stress, a significant contributor to nerve damage in neuropathy[3].

Effects on Neuropathy

- **Pain Reduction**: Omega-3 supplementation has been shown to reduce neuropathic pain by decreasing inflammation and oxidative stress. Studies have demonstrated its effectiveness in alleviating pain and improving quality of life in individuals with neuropathy[1].

- **Improved Sensory Function**: By promoting nerve regeneration and reducing oxidative damage, omega-3 fatty acids help improve sensory and motor functions in individuals with neuropathy[4].
- **Prevention of Neuropathy Progression**: Regular supplementation with omega-3 fatty acids can prevent the progression of neuropathy by maintaining adequate anti-inflammatory and antioxidant defenses[2].

Dosages

The optimal dosage of omega-3 fatty acids for neuropathy varies, but studies suggest that doses ranging from **1 to 3 grams per day** of combined EPA and DHA are generally safe and effective[1]. It is advisable to start with a lower dose and gradually increase it to monitor tolerance and effectiveness. Consulting with a healthcare provider before starting supplementation is recommended to tailor the dosage to individual needs and conditions[1].

Conclusion

Omega-3 fatty acids, through their anti-inflammatory, antioxidant, and neuroprotective properties, offer promising therapeutic benefits for neuropathy. Their mechanisms of action contribute to pain reduction, improved nerve function, and prevention of neuropathy progression. While more research is needed to establish optimal dosages, current evidence supports the potential of omega-3 fatty acids as valuable supplements in managing neuropathy.

Peppermint

Peppermint (Mentha piperita) is a hybrid mint, a cross between watermint and spearmint, known for its distinctive aroma and medicinal properties. It has been traditionally used for various ailments, including digestive issues, headaches, and muscle pain. Recent studies have explored its potential benefits for neuropathy.

Compounds Derived from Peppermint

- **Menthol**: The primary active compound in peppermint oil, known for its cooling and analgesic properties[1].
- **Menthone**: Another significant component that contributes to the analgesic and anti-inflammatory effects of peppermint[1].
- **Flavonoids**: Peppermint contains flavonoids such as luteolin and hesperidin, which have antioxidant and anti-inflammatory properties[2].
- **Rosmarinic Acid**: A phenolic compound with strong antioxidant and anti-inflammatory effects[2].

Mechanisms of Action

- **Analgesic Effects**: Menthol activates transient receptor potential (TRP) channels, particularly TRPM8, which are involved in the sensation of cold and pain relief. This activation leads to a cooling sensation and analgesic effects, helping to alleviate neuropathic pain[1].
- **Anti-inflammatory Properties**: The flavonoids and rosmarinic acid in peppermint reduce inflammation by inhibiting the production of pro-inflammatory cytokines. This helps in mitigating the inflammatory processes associated with neuropathy[2].
- **Antioxidant Activity**: Peppermint's antioxidant compounds, such as flavonoids and rosmarinic acid, scavenge free radicals and reduce oxidative stress, which is a significant contributor to nerve damage in neuropathy[2].
- **Improved Blood Flow**: Menthol has vasodilatory effects, which improve blood flow to the affected areas, enhancing nutrient and oxygen delivery to damaged nerves[1].

Effects on Neuropathy

- **Pain Reduction**: Peppermint oil, particularly its menthol component, has been shown to reduce neuropathic pain by providing a cooling sensation and blocking pain signals[1].
- **Improved Sensory Function**: By reducing inflammation and oxidative stress, peppermint helps improve sensory and motor functions in individuals with neuropathy[2].
- **Enhanced Nerve Regeneration**: The improved blood flow and antioxidant properties of peppermint support nerve repair and regeneration[2].

Dosages

The optimal dosage of peppermint for managing neuropathy varies, but studies suggest that topical application of peppermint oil containing **5-10% menthol** is generally safe and effective[1]. For oral supplementation, doses ranging from **200 to 400 mg per day** of peppermint oil capsules are commonly used[3]. It is advisable to start with a lower dose and gradually increase it to monitor tolerance and effectiveness. Consulting with a healthcare provider before starting supplementation is recommended to tailor the dosage to individual needs and conditions[3].

Conclusion

Peppermint, through its active compounds such as menthol, flavonoids, and rosmarinic acid, offers significant therapeutic benefits for neuropathy. Its mechanisms of action, including analgesic, anti-inflammatory, and antioxidant properties, contribute to pain reduction, improved sensory function, and enhanced nerve regeneration. While more research is needed to establish optimal dosages and long-term safety, current evidence supports the potential of peppermint as a valuable supplement in managing neuropathy.

Plantain (Plantago major)

Plantago major, commonly known as **plantain** (not to be confused with the banana-like fruit), is a perennial herb widely recognized for its medicinal properties. Traditionally used for wound healing and inflammation, plantain may offer potential benefits for neuropathy.

Compounds and Ingredients

Plantain is rich in bioactive compounds that contribute to its therapeutic effects:

- **Iridoid Glycosides**: Primarily **aucubin** and **catalpol**, known for anti-inflammatory and neuroprotective properties (Samuelsen, 2000).

- **Phenylethanoids**: Such as **acteoside** and **isoacteoside**, exhibiting antioxidant and anti-inflammatory activities (Gálvez et al., 2005).

- **Flavonoids**: Including **apigenin, luteolin**, and **baicalein**, which have antioxidant effects (Ji et al., 2012).

- **Polysaccharides**: Contributing to immunomodulatory activities (Paul et al., 2011).

- **Tannins**: With astringent properties that may reduce inflammation.

- **Vitamins and Minerals**: Contains vitamin K, vitamin C, calcium, and zinc, supporting overall health.

Mechanism of Action

Plantain's potential effects on neuropathy can be attributed to several mechanisms:

- **Anti-inflammatory Effects**: Iridoid glycosides and flavonoids inhibit the production of pro-inflammatory cytokines (e.g., TNF-α, IL-1β) and enzymes like COX-2, reducing inflammation that can exacerbate neuropathic pain (Samuelsen, 2000).

- **Antioxidant Activity**: Phenylethanoids and flavonoids scavenge free radicals, decreasing oxidative stress that damages nerve cells (Gálvez et al., 2005).

- **Neuroprotection**: Compounds like aucubin may protect neurons from degeneration by inhibiting apoptotic pathways (Zhang et al., 2011).

- **Immune Modulation**: Polysaccharides enhance immune function by stimulating macrophage activity, potentially aiding in tissue repair (Paul et al., 2011).

- **Wound Healing Properties**: Facilitates tissue regeneration, which might benefit nerve healing processes (Chiang et al., 2002).

Effects on Neuropathy

While direct clinical studies on plantain specifically for neuropathy are limited, the herb's pharmacological actions suggest potential benefits:

- **Pain Reduction**: Anti-inflammatory and analgesic effects may alleviate neuropathic pain.

- **Nerve Repair and Protection**: Antioxidant and neuroprotective properties support nerve regeneration and prevent further damage.

- **Symptom Relief**: Reduction in inflammation and oxidative stress may lessen symptoms like tingling and numbness.

Doses and Administration

There is no standardized dosage of plantain for neuropathy, but general recommendations include:

- **Tea**: Steep 1-2 teaspoons of dried plantain leaves in a cup of hot water for 10-15 minutes. Consume 2-3 times daily.

- **Tincture**: 2-4 ml of plantain tincture (1:5 in 25% alcohol) taken 2-3 times daily.

- **Capsules/Tablets**: Standardized extracts may be available, with dosages according to manufacturer instructions.

- **Topical Application**: Plantain ointments or salves applied to affected areas may help with localized pain.

Safety and Precautions

- **Allergies**: Individuals allergic to plantain species or the Plantaginaceae family should avoid use.

- **Drug Interactions**: May interact with lithium, diuretics, or blood sugar medications. Consult a healthcare provider before use (Samuelsen, 2000).

- **Pregnancy and Lactation**: Safety is not well-established; use cautiously under professional guidance.

- **Contamination Concerns**: Ensure plantain is sourced from areas free of pesticides and pollutants.

History of Use

- **Traditional Medicine**: Used for centuries across Europe, Asia, and North America.

- **Medicinal Uses**:

- *Wound Healing*: Applied to cuts, insect bites, and skin inflammations (Chiang et al., 2002).

- *Anti-inflammatory*: Used to treat respiratory infections, digestive issues, and inflammatory conditions.

- *Diuretic and Expectorant*: Employed in remedies for urinary tract infections and coughs.

- **Cultural Significance**: Known as "the mother of herbs" in some cultures due to its wide-ranging applications.

Conclusion

Plantain (*Plantago major*) exhibits anti-inflammatory, antioxidant, and neuroprotective properties that may offer benefits for individuals with neuropathy. While historical use and pharmacological studies are promising, clinical trials specifically investigating plantain's efficacy for neuropathy are needed. Individuals considering plantain as a complementary treatment should consult healthcare professionals to ensure safety and appropriate usage. Continued research is warranted to fully understand its therapeutic potential and establish evidence-based guidelines.

Poria

Poria cocos, also known as Wolfiporia extensa or **Fu Ling** in Traditional Chinese Medicine (TCM), is a fungus widely used in herbal remedies across Asia. For centuries, Poria has been valued for its diuretic, sedative, and tonic properties. Recent interest has turned towards its potential therapeutic effects on neuropathy—a condition resulting from damaged nerves, often causing weakness, numbness, and pain, typically in the hands and feet.

History of Use

Poria has been a staple in TCM for over 2,000 years. Historical texts, such as the *Shennong Ben Cao Jing* (Divine Farmer's Materia Medica), classify Poria as a superior herb with the ability to nourish the heart and spleen, calm the mind, and promote urination (Bensky & Gamble, 1993). Traditionally, it has been used to address conditions like edema, insomnia, and digestive issues.

Bioactive Compounds and Ingredients

Poria contains several bioactive constituents that contribute to its medicinal properties:

- **Polysaccharides**: Including beta-glucans, which are believed to modulate immune responses and exhibit neuroprotective effects (Zhang et al., 2019).

- **Triterpenoids**: Such as pachymic acid, dehydrotumulosic acid, and eburicoic acid, known for anti-inflammatory and antioxidant activities (Chen et al., 2018).

- **Ergosterol**: A precursor to vitamin D2, with potential antioxidant properties (Li et al., 2014).

Mechanism of Action

The therapeutic potential of Poria in neuropathy may be attributed to the following mechanisms:

- **Anti-inflammatory Effects**: Chronic inflammation is a key contributor to neuropathic pain. Triterpenoids in Poria have been shown to inhibit pro-inflammatory cytokines and mediators, potentially reducing inflammation in nerve tissues (Chen et al., 2018).

- **Antioxidant Activity**: Oxidative stress damages neurons and exacerbates neuropathy. The polysaccharides and triterpenoids in Poria exhibit antioxidant properties that may protect nerve cells from oxidative damage (Zhang et al., 2019).

- **Immune Modulation**: Poria polysaccharides may modulate immune responses, which is significant since autoimmune reactions can contribute to certain types of neuropathy (Wang et al., 2017).

- **Neurotrophic Effects**: Some studies suggest that Poria extracts can promote nerve growth factor (NGF) expression, aiding in nerve repair and regeneration (Liu et al., 2016).

Effects on Neuropathy

While direct clinical studies on Poria's effects on neuropathy are limited, preclinical research provides insights:

- **Animal Studies**: A study by Liu et al. (2016) demonstrated that Poria polysaccharides improved peripheral nerve regeneration in rats with sciatic nerve crush injuries.

- **In vitro Research**: Zhang et al. (2019) found that Poria polysaccharides protected neurons from oxidative stress-induced apoptosis in cell cultures, suggesting potential neuroprotective benefits.

- **Adjunct Therapy**: In TCM, Poria is often used in combination with other herbs for synergistic effects. Some formulations have been studied for diabetic neuropathy with positive outcomes (Li et al., 2015).

Dosing Considerations

Dosage of Poria can vary based on the form and the specific health condition:

- **Traditional Use**: In TCM, typical doses range from 9 to 15 grams of the dried fungus per day, decocted in water (Bensky & Gamble, 1993).

- **Extracts**: Standardized extracts may vary in concentration. It's crucial to follow manufacturer guidelines and consult a healthcare professional before use.

- **Safety**: Poria is generally considered safe with low toxicity. However, high doses may cause gastrointestinal discomfort (Chen et al., 2018).

Different Types and Best Form

Poria is available in several forms:

- **Whole Dried Sclerotium**: Used in traditional decoctions.

- **Powdered Extracts**: Concentrated forms standardized to specific polysaccharide or triterpenoid content.

- **Capsules and Tablets**: For convenience and accurate dosing.

- **Poria Derivatives**: Such as fermented Poria extracts, which may have enhanced bioavailability.

Best Form:

- **Standardized Extracts**: May offer a higher concentration of active compounds, ensuring consistency and potency (Li et al., 2015).

- **Combination Formulas**: In some cases, Poria is more effective when combined with other herbs that support nerve health.

Conclusion

Poria cocos exhibits bioactive properties that may offer therapeutic benefits for neuropathy through anti-inflammatory, antioxidant, immune-modulating, and neurotrophic mechanisms. While historical use and preclinical studies are promising, clinical trials are necessary to fully establish efficacy and safety in neuropathy patients. Individuals interested in Poria supplementation should consult healthcare professionals to determine appropriate forms and dosing.

Quercetin

Quercetin is a natural flavonoid found abundantly in fruits, vegetables, leaves, and grains. It is known for its antioxidant, anti-inflammatory, and neuroprotective properties. Recent research has explored quercetin's potential benefits in managing neuropathy, a condition characterized by nerve damage resulting in pain, tingling, and numbness, often associated with diabetes and other chronic conditions.

Active Ingredients and Compounds

Quercetin itself is the primary active compound—a flavonoid that contributes to the pigmentation in plants. It is present in high concentrations in:

- **Apples**
- **Onions**
- **Berries** (e.g., blueberries, cranberries)
- **Citrus fruits**
- **Leafy greens**
- **Tea**
- **Red wine**

Quercetin is often found in glycoside forms, such as quercetin-3-O-glucoside, where it is bound to sugar molecules, enhancing its bioavailability.

Mechanism of Action

Antioxidant Activity: Quercetin is a potent scavenger of free radicals, reducing oxidative stress—a key factor in nerve damage associated with neuropathy.

Anti-inflammatory Effects: It inhibits the production of pro-inflammatory cytokines (e.g., TNF-α, IL-1β, IL-6), reducing inflammation that contributes to nerve pain.

Neuroprotective Properties:

- **Inhibition of Enzymes**: Quercetin inhibits aldose reductase, an enzyme involved in the polyol pathway that converts glucose to sorbitol. In diabetic neuropathy, excess sorbitol accumulation can lead to nerve damage.
- **Mitochondrial Protection**: It helps maintain mitochondrial function in neurons, preserving energy production and cellular health.
- **Apoptosis Prevention**: Quercetin reduces neuronal cell death by inhibiting apoptosis pathways.

Modulation of Ion Channels: It affects calcium and potassium ion channels, which play roles in nerve signal transmission, potentially alleviating neuropathic pain.

History of Use

Quercetin has been part of human diets for centuries through the consumption of fruits and vegetables rich in this flavonoid. Its therapeutic properties have been recognized in traditional medicine systems for treating various ailments:

- **Traditional Chinese Medicine**: Used plants containing quercetin for their anti-inflammatory and antioxidant effects.
- **Ayurveda**: Employed herbal remedies rich in quercetin for managing inflammation and supporting overall health.

Scientific interest in quercetin's medicinal properties increased in the 20th century, leading to numerous studies on its potential health benefits.

Doses

There is no established Recommended Daily Allowance (RDA) for quercetin. However, studies have used varying doses:

- **Supplement Form**: Common doses range from 500 mg to 1,000 mg per day, divided into two or three doses.
- **Dietary Intake**: Typical dietary intake is estimated to be between 5 mg and 40 mg per day, depending on diet.

Note: High doses may cause side effects in some individuals, such as headaches or digestive discomfort. It is essential to consult a healthcare professional before starting supplementation.

Types and How to Supplement

Forms of Quercetin Supplements:

- **Capsules/Tablets**: Standardized doses for convenient intake.
- **Powders**: Can be mixed with liquids or foods.
- **Combination Supplements**: Often combined with vitamin C or bromelain to enhance absorption and efficacy.

Dietary Sources: Increase intake of quercetin through diet by consuming:

- Apples (with skin)
- Onions (red onions have higher quercetin content)
- Berries
- Grapes
- Leafy greens
- Broccoli
- Citrus fruits

Conclusion

Quercetin shows promise as a natural compound for managing neuropathy due to its antioxidant, anti-inflammatory, and neuroprotective properties. While research is ongoing, preliminary studies suggest it may help reduce nerve pain and prevent further nerve damage. Individuals interested in quercetin supplementation should consult healthcare professionals to ensure safety and appropriateness, considering possible interactions with medications and individual health status.

Sumac (Rhus coriaria)

Sumac, scientifically known as **Rhus coriaria**, is a flowering plant that produces deep red berries. It has a rich history of use in cooking, traditional medicine, and as a natural dye. Sumac has been used traditionally for its medicinal properties.

Compounds and Ingredients

Sumac is rich in bioactive compounds that may contribute to its therapeutic effects:

- Polyphenols: Sumac contains high levels of polyphenolic compounds, including gallic acid, methyl gallate, and tannins, which exhibit strong antioxidant properties (Gul et al., 2017).
- Flavonoids: Such as quercetin, kaempferol, and myricetin, known for their anti-inflammatory and antioxidant effects (İlahı et al., 2020).
- Anthocyanins: Pigments responsible for the red coloration of sumac berries, possessing antioxidant activity (Pourahmad et al., 2010).
- Organic Acids: Including malic acid and citric acid, contributing to the sour taste and potential antimicrobial properties (Kosar et al., 2007).
- Essential Oils: Sumac contains volatile oils that may have antimicrobial and anti-inflammatory effects (Mohammadhosseini et al., 2017).

Mechanism of Action

Sumac's potential benefits for neuropathy can be attributed to several mechanisms:

- Antioxidant Activity: The polyphenols and flavonoids in sumac scavenge free radicals, reducing oxidative stress that contributes to nerve damage in neuropathy (Gul et al., 2017).

- Anti-inflammatory Effects: Sumac compounds inhibit the production of pro-inflammatory cytokines (e.g., TNF-α, IL-1β), potentially reducing inflammation around nerves (İlahı et al., 2020).
- Neuroprotective Properties: Antioxidant and anti-inflammatory actions may protect neurons from degeneration and support nerve regeneration (Pourahmad et al., 2010).
- Blood Glucose Regulation: Sumac has been shown to help regulate blood sugar levels, which is significant since uncontrolled diabetes is a common cause of neuropathy (Esmaeili & Yazdanparast, 2004).

Effects on Neuropathy

While direct clinical studies on sumac's effects on neuropathy are limited, the combined pharmacological actions suggest potential benefits:

- Pain Reduction: Anti-inflammatory and analgesic effects may alleviate neuropathic pain.
- Nerve Protection: Antioxidant properties may prevent further nerve damage and support repair processes.
- Symptom Improvement: Reducing inflammation and oxidative stress may lessen symptoms like tingling and numbness.

Doses and Administration

There is no standardized dosage of sumac for neuropathy, but general recommendations include:

- Sumac Spice: Commonly used as a culinary spice; however, therapeutic doses may differ from dietary amounts.
- Extracts and Supplements: Sumac extracts standardized for polyphenol content are available. Typical doses in studies range from 500 mg to 3 grams per day, but it's essential to follow product-specific guidelines or consult a healthcare provider (Jalali et al., 2020).
- Tea Infusion: Preparing a tea by steeping 1-2 teaspoons of dried sumac berries in hot water for 10-15 minutes, consumed 1-2 times daily.

Safety and Precautions

- Species Identification: Ensure the use of non-toxic species (*Rhus coriaria*) and avoid poisonous varieties like poison sumac (*Toxicodendron vernix*), which can cause severe allergic reactions.
- Allergies: Individuals allergic to plants in the Anacardiaceae family (e.g., cashews, mangoes) should exercise caution.
- Pregnancy and Lactation: Safety has not been established; consult a healthcare provider before use.
- Drug Interactions: Sumac may interact with medications, including antidiabetic drugs and blood thinners. Professional guidance is recommended.

History of Use

Sumac has a rich history in traditional medicine:

- Traditional Practices: Used in Middle Eastern, Mediterranean, and Asian cultures for its medicinal properties, including as an astringent, antiseptic, and anti-inflammatory agent (Zare et al., 2019).
- Culinary Uses: Employed as a spice to add a tangy flavor to dishes, contributing antioxidants to the diet.
- Folk Remedies: Traditionally used to treat ailments like diarrhea, sore throats, and infections due to its antimicrobial properties.

Conclusion

Sumac (*Rhus coriaria*) exhibits antioxidant and anti-inflammatory properties that may offer benefits for individuals with neuropathy. While traditional uses and preliminary studies are promising, clinical trials specifically investigating sumac's efficacy for neuropathy are necessary to substantiate these claims. Individuals considering sumac as a complementary treatment should consult healthcare professionals to ensure safety and appropriate usage. Continued research is warranted to fully understand sumac's therapeutic potential and establish evidence-based guidelines.

TB-500

TB-500, also known as Thymosin Beta-4 (TB4), is a synthetic peptide that has garnered attention for its potential therapeutic benefits, particularly in tissue repair and regeneration.

Compounds Derived from TB-500

- **Thymosin Beta-4 (TB4)**: The primary active compound in TB-500, TB4 is a naturally occurring peptide that plays a crucial role in tissue repair and regeneration[1].
- **TB-500**: A synthetic version of TB4, designed to mimic its effects and enhance its stability and bioavailability[2].

Mechanisms of Action

- **Promotion of Nerve Regeneration**: TB-500 promotes the regeneration of nerve cells by upregulating the expression of genes involved in cell migration, differentiation, and survival. It enhances the repair of damaged nerves, which is crucial for alleviating neuropathic pain[3].
- **Anti-inflammatory Effects**: TB-500 reduces inflammation by modulating the activity of pro-inflammatory cytokines and pathways. This helps in mitigating the inflammatory processes associated with neuropathy[1].
- **Angiogenesis and Vasculogenesis**: TB-500 stimulates the formation of new blood vessels (angiogenesis) and the repair of existing ones (vasculogenesis). Improved blood flow to damaged nerves enhances nutrient and oxygen delivery, promoting nerve repair and reducing neuropathic pain[2].
- **Reduction of Oxidative Stress**: TB-500 has antioxidant properties that help in reducing oxidative stress, a significant contributor to nerve damage in neuropathy[3].

Effects on Neuropathy

- **Pain Reduction**: TB-500 has been shown to reduce neuropathic pain by promoting nerve regeneration and reducing inflammation. Studies on rodent models have demonstrated its effectiveness in decreasing hypersensitivity and alleviating pain behaviors[3].

- **Improved Sensory Function**: By enhancing nerve repair and reducing oxidative damage, TB-500 helps improve sensory and motor functions in individuals with neuropathy[1].
- **Prevention of Neuropathy Progression**: Regular use of TB-500 can prevent the progression of neuropathy by maintaining adequate blood flow and reducing inflammatory and oxidative damage to nerves[2].

Dosages

The optimal dosage of TB-500 for managing neuropathy varies, but studies suggest that doses ranging from **2 to 5 mg per week** are generally safe and effective[2]. It is advisable to start with a lower dose and gradually increase it to monitor tolerance and effectiveness. TB-500 is typically administered via subcutaneous or intramuscular injections. Consulting with a healthcare provider before starting supplementation is recommended to tailor the dosage to individual needs and conditions[2].

Conclusion

TB-500, through its nerve regeneration, anti-inflammatory, and angiogenic properties, offers promising therapeutic benefits for neuropathy. Its mechanisms of action contribute to pain reduction, improved sensory function, and prevention of neuropathy progression. While more research is needed to establish optimal dosages and long-term safety, current evidence supports the potential of TB-500 as a valuable treatment option for managing neuropathy.

THC (Marijuana)

Tetrahydrocannabinol (THC), the primary psychoactive compound in cannabis, has been studied for its potential benefits in treating neuropathic pain. This drug is still illegal in many states. Talk to your doctor about a prescription.

Compounds and Ingredients

THC is one of over 100 cannabinoids found in the cannabis plant. The primary compounds in THC include:

- **Delta-9-Tetrahydrocannabinol (Δ9-THC)**: The main psychoactive component responsible for the "high" associated with cannabis use.
- **Cannabidiol** (CBD): A non-psychoactive cannabinoid that may enhance the therapeutic effects of THC while mitigating some of its psychoactive effects.
- **Terpenes**: Aromatic compounds that contribute to the plant's scent and may have therapeutic properties.

Mechanism of Action

- Interaction with Cannabinoid Receptors: THC binds to cannabinoid receptors (CB1 and CB2) in the central and peripheral nervous systems. CB1 receptors are primarily located in the brain and spinal cord, while CB2 receptors are found in immune cells and peripheral tissues. Activation of these receptors modulates pain perception and inflammation (Pertwee, 2008).
- Modulation of Neurotransmitter Release: THC influences the release of neurotransmitters such as dopamine, serotonin, and glutamate, which play roles in pain signaling and mood regulation (Mackie, 2008).
- Anti-inflammatory Effects: THC reduces the production of pro-inflammatory cytokines and increases the release of anti-inflammatory cytokines, potentially reducing inflammation around nerves (Nagarkatti et al., 2009).

- Neuroprotective Properties: THC has antioxidant properties that protect neurons from oxidative stress and apoptosis, which can contribute to nerve damage (Hampson et al., 1998).

Effects on Neuropathy

Research suggests that THC may offer several benefits for individuals with neuropathy:
- Pain Relief: THC's interaction with cannabinoid receptors can reduce pain perception and alleviate neuropathic pain (Wallace et al., 2015).
- Reduction of Inflammation: Anti-inflammatory effects may decrease nerve inflammation and associated symptoms.
- Improvement in Sleep and Mood: By modulating neurotransmitter release, THC may improve sleep quality and reduce anxiety and depression, which are common in individuals with chronic pain (Russo, 2008).

Doses and Administration

The appropriate dose of THC can vary based on individual factors and the method of administration:

- Inhalation: Smoking or vaporizing cannabis allows for rapid onset of effects. Typical doses range from 2.5 to 10 mg of THC per session.
- Oral Consumption: Edibles and tinctures provide longer-lasting effects but have a delayed onset. Doses typically range from 5 to 20 mg of THC.
- Topical Application: THC-infused creams and balms can be applied directly to affected areas for localized relief.

Safety and Precautions

- Side Effects: THC can cause side effects such as dizziness, dry mouth, increased heart rate, and impaired cognitive function. Higher doses may increase the risk of adverse effects.
- Tolerance and Dependence: Regular use of THC can lead to tolerance, requiring higher doses to achieve the same effects. There is also a potential for dependence and withdrawal symptoms.
- Legal Considerations: The legal status of THC varies by region. It is important to be aware of local laws and regulations regarding cannabis use.

History of Use

Cannabis has been used for medicinal purposes for thousands of years:

- Ancient Use: Historical records indicate that cannabis was used in ancient China, India, and Egypt for its analgesic and anti-inflammatory properties (Russo, 2007).
- Modern Medicine: In the 19th and early 20th centuries, cannabis extracts were commonly used in Western medicine for pain relief and other ailments. However, its use declined due to legal restrictions and the development of synthetic pharmaceuticals.
- Recent Resurgence: Interest in medical cannabis has resurged in recent decades, driven by growing evidence of its therapeutic potential and changing legal landscapes.

Conclusion

THC, the primary psychoactive compound in cannabis, exhibits several pharmacological properties that may benefit individuals with neuropathy. Its interaction with cannabinoid receptors, modulation of neurotransmitter release, anti-inflammatory effects, and neuroprotective properties suggest potential for pain relief and improved quality of life. However, further research is needed to fully understand its efficacy and safety. Individuals considering THC for neuropathy should consult healthcare professionals and be aware of legal considerations. Continued research and clinical trials are essential to establish evidence-based guidelines for its use.

Vitamin B12

Vitamin B12, also known as **cobalamin**, is a crucial nutrient for maintaining nerve health and function. Vitamin B12 is a water-soluble vitamin that plays a vital role in the production of red blood cells, DNA synthesis, and the proper functioning of the nervous system[1]. It is found naturally in animal products such as meat, fish, poultry, eggs, and dairy products. Vitamin B12 can also be taken as a dietary supplement or administered via injection for those with deficiencies[1].

Effects on Neuropathy

Neuropathy, particularly peripheral neuropathy, involves damage to the peripheral nerves, leading to symptoms such as pain, tingling, and numbness. Vitamin B12 has shown promise in alleviating these symptoms through several mechanisms:

- **Pain Reduction**: Clinical studies have demonstrated that vitamin B12 can significantly reduce neuropathic pain. It helps alleviate symptoms by promoting myelination, increasing nerve regeneration, and decreasing ectopic nerve firing[2].
- **Improved Nerve Function**: Vitamin B12 is essential for the maintenance of the myelin sheath, the protective covering around nerves. This is particularly beneficial for individuals with diabetic neuropathy, as it helps restore normal nerve activity[2].
- **Neuroprotection**: Vitamin B12 provides neuroprotective effects by safeguarding nerve cells from further damage. This is achieved through its role in DNA synthesis and repair, as well as its antioxidant properties[2].

Active Compounds and Mechanisms of Action

The beneficial effects of vitamin B12 on neuropathy are primarily attributed to its role in cellular metabolism and its neuroprotective properties. Here's how vitamin B12 and its related compounds work:

- **Methylcobalamin**: This is the active form of vitamin B12 that is directly involved in the synthesis of methionine from homocysteine. Methionine is crucial for the production of S-adenosylmethionine (SAMe), a compound involved in methylation reactions essential for DNA repair and myelin synthesis[3].

- **Adenosylcobalamin**: Another active form of vitamin B12, adenosylcobalamin, is involved in the conversion of methylmalonyl-CoA to succinyl-CoA, a critical step in the production of energy within cells. This process is vital for maintaining the health and function of nerve cells[3].
- **Myelin Synthesis**: Vitamin B12 is essential for the formation and maintenance of the myelin sheath. Myelin is the protective covering around nerves that ensures the rapid transmission of nerve impulses. Deficiency in vitamin B12 can lead to demyelination, resulting in nerve damage and neuropathy[4].
- **Reduction of Homocysteine Levels**: Elevated homocysteine levels are associated with an increased risk of neuropathy. Vitamin B12 helps convert homocysteine to methionine, thereby reducing homocysteine levels and protecting nerves from damage[4].
- **Antioxidant Activity**: Vitamin B12 has antioxidant properties that help neutralize free radicals, reducing oxidative stress and protecting nerve cells from damage[4].

Conclusion

Vitamin B12 is a vital nutrient with significant potential benefits for managing neuropathy. Its role in myelin synthesis, DNA repair, and reduction of oxidative stress makes it a valuable supplement for individuals suffering from neuropathic pain. However, it is important to use vitamin B12 under the guidance of a healthcare professional to ensure safety and efficacy.

Vitamin B6

Vitamin B6, also known as pyridoxine, is a water-soluble vitamin that plays a crucial role in numerous physiological functions, including amino acid metabolism, neurotransmitter synthesis, and hemoglobin production. Its impact on neuropathy, particularly peripheral neuropathy, has been widely studied.

Compounds Derived from Vitamin B6

- **Pyridoxine**: The most common form of Vitamin B6 found in supplements and fortified foods.
- **Pyridoxal 5'-phosphate (PLP)**: The active form of Vitamin B6 that acts as a coenzyme in various enzymatic reactions.
- **Pyridoxamine**: Another form of Vitamin B6 that is involved in the metabolism of amino acids and neurotransmitters[1].

Mechanisms of Action

- **Neurotransmitter Synthesis**: Vitamin B6 is essential for the synthesis of neurotransmitters such as serotonin, dopamine, and gamma-aminobutyric acid (GABA). These neurotransmitters play a critical role in nerve function and pain modulation[1].
- **Homocysteine Metabolism**: Vitamin B6 helps in the conversion of homocysteine to cysteine. Elevated levels of homocysteine are associated with neurotoxicity and can contribute to neuropathy[2].
- **Anti-inflammatory Effects**: Vitamin B6 has anti-inflammatory properties that help reduce inflammation, which is a key factor in the progression of neuropathy[3].
- **Antioxidant Properties**: Vitamin B6 acts as an antioxidant, protecting nerve cells from oxidative stress and damage[3].

Effects on Neuropathy

- **Pain Reduction**: Vitamin B6 supplementation has been shown to reduce neuropathic pain. This is primarily due to its role in neurotransmitter synthesis and its anti-inflammatory effects[1].
- **Improved Nerve Function**: By supporting neurotransmitter synthesis and reducing oxidative stress, Vitamin B6 helps in the repair and

regeneration of damaged nerves, leading to improved sensory and motor functions[2].

- **Prevention of Neuropathy Progression**: Regular supplementation with Vitamin B6 can prevent the progression of neuropathy by maintaining adequate levels of neurotransmitters and reducing inflammatory and oxidative damage to nerves[3].

Dosages

The optimal dosage of Vitamin B6 for neuropathy varies. The recommended dietary allowance (RDA) for adults is **1.3 to 2 mg per day**[4]. However, higher doses are often used in clinical settings to manage neuropathy. Doses ranging from **50 to 100 mg per day** have been found to be effective[4]. It is important to note that excessive intake of Vitamin B6 (above 200 mg per day) can lead to toxicity and cause sensory neuropathy[5]. Therefore, it is advisable to consult with a healthcare provider before starting supplementation to tailor the dosage to individual needs and conditions[5].

Conclusion

Vitamin B6, through its roles in neurotransmitter synthesis, homocysteine metabolism, and its anti-inflammatory and antioxidant properties, offers promising therapeutic benefits for neuropathy. Its mechanisms of action contribute to pain reduction, improved nerve function, and prevention of neuropathy progression. While more research is needed to establish optimal dosages, current evidence supports the potential of Vitamin B6 as a valuable supplement in managing neuropathy.

White Mulberry

White mulberry (Morus alba) is a deciduous tree native to China, widely cultivated for its leaves, which are the primary food source for silkworms. Beyond its significance in the silk industry, white mulberry has been used in traditional medicine for centuries. Recent research has explored its potential benefits for neuropathy—a condition characterized by nerve damage resulting in pain, tingling, and numbness, often associated with diabetes and other chronic diseases.

Active Ingredients and Compounds

White mulberry contains a variety of bioactive compounds contributing to its medicinal properties:

- **1-Deoxynojirimycin (DNJ):** A potent α-glucosidase inhibitor that helps regulate blood sugar levels by slowing carbohydrate digestion and absorption.
- **Flavonoids:** Such as quercetin, kaempferol, and rutin, which possess antioxidant and anti-inflammatory properties.
- **Phenolic Acids:** Including gallic acid and caffeic acid, known for their antioxidant activities.
- **Alkaloids and Coumarins:** Contribute to overall health benefits, including vasodilation and neuroprotection.
- **Polysaccharides:** May enhance immune function and exhibit neuroprotective effects.

Mechanism of Action

The potential benefits of white mulberry for neuropathy are attributed to several mechanisms:

- **Blood Sugar Regulation:** DNJ inhibits enzymes responsible for carbohydrate digestion, leading to lower postprandial blood glucose levels. Maintaining stable blood sugar is crucial for preventing diabetic neuropathy.

- **Antioxidant Effects:** Flavonoids and phenolic acids scavenge free radicals, reducing oxidative stress—a key factor in nerve damage and neuropathy progression.
- **Anti-inflammatory Properties:** White mulberry extracts can suppress pro-inflammatory cytokines, reducing inflammation associated with nerve damage.
- **Neuroprotective Effects:** Studies suggest that white mulberry compounds may protect neurons from apoptosis (cell death) and promote nerve regeneration.
- **Improved Microcirculation:** By enhancing blood flow, white mulberry may improve oxygen and nutrient delivery to damaged nerves.

History of Use

- **Traditional Chinese Medicine (TCM):** White mulberry, known as "Sang Ye," has been used for over 3,000 years. It is employed to treat fever, headaches, eye infections, and to promote liver health.
- **Diabetes Management:** Historically used to control blood sugar levels, thereby preventing complications like neuropathy.
- **Other Cultures:** Used in various traditional remedies across Asia and Europe for ailments such as hypertension, arthritis, and infections.

Doses

- **Capsules/Tablets:** Common dosages range from **500 mg to 1,000 mg**, taken **two to three times daily** before meals.
- **Tea:** Steep **1–2 teaspoons** of dried mulberry leaves in hot water for **5–10 minutes**. Consume **1–3 times daily**.
- **Extracts:** Liquid extracts can be taken as per manufacturer's instructions, typically **30–60 drops** in water or juice, taken **2–3 times daily**.

Types and How to Supplement

- **Mulberry Leaf Supplements:** Available in capsules, tablets, and powdered forms. Standardized extracts ensure consistent levels of active compounds like DNJ.
- **Mulberry Leaf Tea:** Dried leaves brewed into a tea, offering a mild and natural way to consume the herb.
- **Liquid Extracts/Tinctures:** Concentrated forms that can be added to beverages for easy consumption.
- **Combination Supplements:** Some products combine white mulberry with other herbs known to support nerve health.

Supplementation Tips:

- **Quality Assurance:** Choose products from reputable manufacturers that offer third-party testing for purity and potency.
- **Medical Consultation:** Especially important for individuals taking medications for diabetes, blood pressure, or cholesterol, as white mulberry may enhance the effects of these drugs.
- **Monitor Blood Sugar Levels:** Diabetic patients should closely monitor glucose levels to avoid hypoglycemia.
- **Allergies and Sensitivities:** Be aware of potential allergic reactions; discontinue use if adverse effects occur.

Conclusion

White mulberry (Morus alba) shows promise as a natural supplement for managing neuropathy due to its blood sugar-regulating, antioxidant, anti-inflammatory, and neuroprotective properties. By addressing key factors involved in neuropathy development and progression, it may offer a complementary approach to conventional treatments. However, more extensive clinical research is needed to establish definitive efficacy and safety. Individuals considering white mulberry supplementation should consult healthcare professionals to ensure appropriate usage and to avoid potential interactions with medications.

Sources For diabetes and blood sugar

Understanding type 2 diabetes

1. https://www.mayoclinic.org/diseases-conditions/type-2-diabetes/symptoms-causes/syc-20351193
2. https://my.clevelandclinic.org/health/diseases/21501-type-2-diabetes
3. https://www.health.harvard.edu/diseases-and-conditions/type-2-diabetes-mellitus-a-to-z
4. https://en.m.wikipedia.org/wiki/Type_2_diabetes
5. https://www.hopkinsmedicine.org/health/conditions-and-diseases/diabetes/type-2-diabetes
6. https://www.bing.com/search?q=type+2+diabetes+causes&FORM=bngcht&toWww=1&redig=8ED459573A1242AF90318B10F4A74479
7. https://www.healthline.com/health/diabetes/type-2-diabetes-causes
8. https://www.nhs.uk/conditions/type-2-diabetes/

Understanding type 1 diabetes

1. https://www.bing.com/search?q=type+1+diabetes+definition&FORM=bngcht&FORM=bngcht&toWww=1&redig=D152F7DC7C3B4988ACAA7DF78D3BA1E8
2. https://www.mayoclinic.org/diseases-conditions/type-1-diabetes/symptoms-causes/syc-20353011
3. https://diabetes.org/about-diabetes/type-1
4. https://my.clevelandclinic.org/health/diseases/21500-type-1-diabetes
5. https://my.clevelandclinic.org/health/diseases/21500-type-1-diabetes
6. https://www.bing.com/search?q=type+1+diabetes+vs+type+2+diabetes&FORM=bngcht&toWww=1&redig=1252F5CA68CD4AEE9646A5BD34A2BE4E
7. https://www.buoyhealth.com/learn/type-1-vs-type2-diabetes
8. https://www.healthline.com/health/difference-between-type-1-and-type-2-diabetes
9. https://uvahealth.com/services/diabetes-care/types

Trans Fats

1. https://diabetes.org/food-nutrition/reading-food-labels/fats
2. https://www.freedomfromdiabetes.org/blog/post/trans-fats-and-the-correlation-with-type-2-diabetes/2998
3. https://www.health.harvard.edu/staying-healthy/the-truth-about-fats-bad-and-good
4. https://www.healthline.com/nutrition/why-trans-fats-are-bad
5. https://www.heart.org/en/healthy-living/healthy-eating/eat-smart/fats/trans-fat

Dietary Fiber

1. https://www.cdc.gov/diabetes/healthy-eating/fiber-helps-diabetes.html
2. https://www.webmd.com/diabetes/understanding-carbohydrates-fiber
3. https://www.everydayhealth.com/hs/type-2-diabetes-live-better-guide/fiber-rich-foods-pictures/
4. https://www.eatingwell.com/article/7994446/best-high-fiber-foods-for-diabetes/
5. https://agamatrix.com/blog/high-fiber-foods-diabetes/
6. https://www.shutterstock.com/image-photo/vegan-health-food-concept-high-fibre-743001070

Weight Training

1. https://diabetesstrong.com/how-resistance-training-affects-your-blood-sugar/
2. https://www.healthline.com/health-news/weight-training-can-help-people-with-type-2-diabetes
3. https://diabetes.org/health-wellness/fitness/anaerobic-exercise-diabetes
4. https://www.everydayhealth.com/type-2-diabetes/living-with/weight-lifting-get-strong/
5. https://diatribe.org/exercise/benefits-strength-training-diabetes

Acetyl L Carnitine

1. https://www.nature.com/articles/s41387-018-0017-1.pdf
2. https://diabetesjournals.org/diabetes/article/62/1/1/15263/AcylcarnitinesReflecting-or-Inflicting-Insulin
3. https://www.frontiersin.org/journals/nutrition/articles/10.3389/fnut.2021.748075/pdf
4. https://www.mayoclinic.org/diseases-conditions/diabetic-neuropathy/in-depth/diabetic-neuropathy-and-dietary-supplements/art-20095406
5. https://www.healthline.com/nutrition/l-carnitine
6. https://link.springer.com/article/10.1007/s10787-023-01323-9
7. https://ods.od.nih.gov/factsheets/Carnitine-Consumer/
8. https://diabetesjournals.org/diabetes/article/62/1/1/15263/AcylcarnitinesReflecting-or-Inflicting-Insulin
9. https://www.frontiersin.org/journals/nutrition/articles/10.3389/fnut.2021.748075/pdf
10. https://academic.oup.com/clinchem/article/51/9/1673/5629882

Allulose

1. Cleveland Clinic. (2024). Allulose: What It Is and Side Effects. Retrieved from Cleveland Clinic
2. Diabetes Meal Plans. (2024). Is Allulose Safe for Diabetics? Retrieved from Diabetes Meal Plans
3. The Food Trends. (2024). What is Allulose Made From? Benefits and Uses. Retrieved from The Food Trends
4. WebMD. (2023). Allulose: What to Know. Retrieved from WebMD

Alpha Lipoic Acid

1. https://www.mdpi.com/2072-6643/15/1/18
2. https://www.frontiersin.org/journals/pharmacology/articles/10.3389/fphar.2011.00069/full
3. https://www.mdpi.com/2072-6643/15/16/3634
4. https://www.preventivemedicinedaily.com/diseases-conditions/endocrine/diabetes/alpha-lipoic-acid-for-diabetes-benefits-and-usage/
5. https://diabetesjournals.org/diabetes/article/50/6/1464/11180/The-Antihyperglycemic-Drug-Lipoic-Acid-Stimulates
6. https://www.mdpi.com/openaccess

Apple Cider Vinegar

1. https://diabetesstrong.com/apple-cider-vinegar-diabetes/
2. https://www.diabetes.co.uk/food/apple-cider-vinegar.html
3. https://www.healthline.com/health/type-2-diabetes/apple-cider-vinegar
4. https://diabetesaction.org/article-vinegar
5. https://link.springer.com/content/pdf/10.1186/s12906-021-03351-w.pdf
6. https://www.bing.com/search?q=apple+cider+vinegar+effects+on+blood+sugar+and+diabetes&FORM=bngcht&toWww=1&redig=BAFBDBD4C0414DCF8EC3A7E076F4A416
7. https://www.webmd.com/diet/apple-cider-vinegar-and-your-health

Apple Pectin

1. https://www.healthline.com/nutrition/apple-pectin
2. https://www.verywellhealth.com/the-benefits-of-apple-pectin-89599
3. https://link.springer.com/article/10.1007/s42452-024-05968-1

4. https://draxe.com/nutrition/pectin/
5. https://www.cambridge.org/core/journals/nutrition-research-reviews/article/nutrition-and-health-effects-of-pectin-a-systematic-scoping-review-of-human-intervention-studies/01BF0759F09A2BBC419F333B8B1D4FF9

Anamu

1. https://www.healthline.com/nutrition/anamu
2. https://www.medicinenet.com/anamu/article.htm
3. https://cosmicattitude.com/en/what-is-anamu-properties-and-benefits/
4. https://www.medicinenet.com/what_is_anamu_herb_good_for/article.htm

Arjuna

1. https://www.mdpi.com/1424-8247/16/1/126
2. https://scialert.net/fulltext/?doi=ijp.2010.515.534
3. https://www.organicgyaan.com/blogs/health-nutrition/arjuna-advantages-risks-and-dosage
4. https://www.earthclinic.com/herbs/arjuna.html
5. https://link.springer.com/chapter/10.1007/978-981-19-0027-3_8

Arnica

1. https://academic.oup.com/jpp/article-abstract/69/8/925/6127789
2. https://www.mdpi.com/2305-6320/8/10/58
3. https://www.gaiaherbs.com/blogs/seeds-of-knowledge/arnica
4. https://link.springer.com/chapter/10.1007/978-981-19-6080-2_4
5. https://link.springer.com/article/10.1007/s11101-023-09884-x
6. https://academic.oup.com/journals/pages/open_access/funder_policies/chorus/standard_publication_model%29
7. https://fjps.springeropen.com/articles/10.1186/s43094-022-00443-3

Astragalus

1. WebMD - Astragalus: Health Benefits, Uses, Dosage, and More
2. Healthline - Astragalus (Huáng Qí): Benefits, Side Effects and Dosage
3. Memorial Sloan Kettering Cancer Center - Astragalus

4. Medical News Today - Astragalus: Benefits, Side Effects, and
   Frequently Asked Questions
5. Frontiers in Pharmacology - A Review of the Pharmacological Action
   of Astragalus Polysaccharide

Barberry

1. https://www.healthline.com/nutrition/barberries
2. https://www.verywellhealth.com/barberry-berberis-vulgaris-what-you-
   need-to-know-89546
3. https://www.webmd.com/vitamins-and-supplements/health-benefits-of-
   barberries
4. https://www.everydayhealth.com/type-2-diabetes/potential-benefits-
   berberine-type-2-diabetes/
5. https://www.healthline.com/nutrition/barberries
6. https://www.verywellhealth.com/barberry-berberis-vulgaris-what-you-
   need-to-know-89546

Bearberry

1. https://www.mdpi.com/1424-8247/17/1/7
2. https://link.springer.com/article/10.1007/s43450-021-00159-0
3. https://www.mdpi.com/2079-7737/12/7/973
4. https://link.springer.com/article/10.1007/s43555-024-00040-w
5. https://www.frontiersin.org/journals/pharmacology/articles/10.3389/fph
   ar.2022.1015045/full

Beech

1. https://fjps.springeropen.com/articles/10.1186/s43094-022-00443-3
2. https://www.frontiersin.org/journals/pharmacology/articles/10.3389/fph
   ar.2021.692566/full
3. https://link.springer.com/article/10.1007/s40495-021-00255-8
4. https://nutritionandmetabolism.biomedcentral.com/articles/10.1186/s1
   2986-024-00829-5

Berberine

1. https://link.springer.com/article/10.1007/s43450-021-00159-0

2. https://www.mdpi.com/1424-8247/17/1/7

3. https://www.healthline.com/nutrition/berberine-diabetes

4. https://link.springer.com/article/10.1007/s00894-024-06060-6

5. https://www.frontiersin.org/journals/endocrinology/articles/10.3389/fendo.2021.609134/full

Beth Root

1. https://nutritionandmetabolism.biomedcentral.com/articles/10.1186/s12986-019-0421-0
2. https://fjps.springeropen.com/articles/10.1186/s43094-022-00443-3
3. https://www.mdpi.com/1648-9144/60/3/394

Bilberry

1. https://www.frontiersin.org/journals/pharmacology/articles/10.3389/fphar.2022.909914/full
2. https://restorativemedicine.org/library/monographs/bilberry/
3. https://altmedrev.com/wp-content/uploads/2019/02/v6-5-500.pdf
4. https://www.mdpi.com/1420-3049/25/7/1653
5. https://link.springer.com/article/10.1007/s13105-020-00739-z
6. https://link.springer.com/article/10.1007/s11892-018-1042-0
7. https://link.springer.com/article/10.1007/s40495-021-00255-8
8. https://link.springer.com/article/10.1007/s43555-024-00040-w

Bitter Melon

1. https://www.webmd.com/diabetes/bitter-melon-help-diabetes
2. https://www.medicalnewstoday.com/articles/317724
3. https://www.eatingwell.com/article/7966460/what-is-bitter-melon-and-can-it-help-you-manage-your-blood-sugar/
4. https://www.healthline.com/health/diabetes/bitter-melon-and-diabetes
5. https://www.nature.com/articles/nutd201442.pdf
6. https://openaccesspub.org/article/2019/ijn-23-4737.pdf
7. https://nutritionj.biomedcentral.com/articles/10.1186/1475-2891-14-13
8. https://www.cambridge.org/core/journals/british-journal-of-nutrition/article/antidiabetic-and-hypoglycaemic-effects-of-momordica-charantia-bitter-melon-a-mini-review/178D6AD854F78BC646ED1D761A394D6D

Bitter Root

1. https://openaccesspub.org/article/2019/ijn-23-4737.pdf
2. https://www.frontiersin.org/journals/pharmacology/articles/10.3389/fph
   ar.2022.904643/full
3. https://www.nature.com/articles/nutd201442.pdf
4. https://discover.texasrealfood.com/roots-of-wellness/bitter-melon
5. https://bmcplantbiol.biomedcentral.com/articles/10.1186/s12870-024-
   05688-z
6. https://fjps.springeropen.com/articles/10.1186/s43094-022-00443-3
7. https://link.springer.com/article/10.1007/s11892-018-1042-0
8. https://link.springer.com/article/10.1007/s40200-021-00853-9

Black Seed Oil

1. https://www.healthline.com/health/black-seed-oil-for-diabetes
2. https://www.diabeticinformed.com/power-black-seed-oil-diabetes/
3. https://www.organicsnature.co/blogs/news/black-seed-oil-for-diabetes-
   and-blood-sugar
4. https://health.clevelandclinic.org/black-seed-oil
5. https://www.lalpathlabs.com/blog/benefits-of-black-seed-oil-in-
   diabetes/
6. https://www.foodnavigator-asia.com/Article/2021/06/22/RCT-supports-
   black-seed-oil-s-blood-sugar-benefits
7. https://www.medicalnewstoday.com/articles/322948

Blue Flag

1. https://diabetesjournals.org/spectrum/article/27/2/100/32064/Novel-
   Agents-for-the-Treatment-of-Type-2-Diabetes
2. https://www.jabfm.org/content/37/3/372
3. https://diabetesjournals.org/clinical/article/23/2/64/1380/Oral-Agents-
   for-Type-2-Diabetes-An-Update

Bromelain

1. https://www.medicalnewstoday.com/articles/323783
2. https://www.webmd.com/vitamins/ai/ingredientmono-895/bromelain
3. https://scientificdiet.org/2024/03/pineapple-and-diabetes-a-sweet-
   surprise/
4. https://pubs.rsc.org/en/content/articlelanding/2023/fo/d3fo01060k

5. https://www.thediabetescouncil.com/pineapple-juice-and-diabetes-benefits-and-side-effects/
6. https://www.webmd.com/vitamins/ai/ingredientmono-895/bromelain
7. https://www.mdpi.com/2072-6643/16/13/2060
8. https://diabetesjournals.org/care/article/46/9/1681/153434/Artificial-Sweeteners-and-Risk-of-Type-2-Diabetes

Cayenne Pepper

1. https://beatdiabetesapp.in/cayenne-pepper-for-diabetes/
2. https://diabetesjournals.org/care/article/26/4/1277/23631/Systematic-Review-of-Herbs-and-Dietary-Supplements
3. https://dmsjournal.biomedcentral.com/articles/10.1186/s13098-017-0254-9

Cats Claw

1. https://facty.com/lifestyle/wellness/the-remarkable-health-benefits-of-cats-claw/
2. https://www.genemedics.com/cats-claw-bark
3. https://clinphytoscience.springeropen.com/articles/10.1186/s40816-021-00332-x
4. https://www.healthline.com/nutrition/cats-claw
5. https://www.nccih.nih.gov/health/cats-claw
6. https://draxe.com/nutrition/cats-claw/

Ceylon Cinnamon

1. https://www.webmd.com/vitamins/ai/ingredientmono-330/ceylon-cinnamon
2. https://draxe.com/nutrition/ceylon-cinnamon-benefits/
3. https://www.healthline.com/nutrition/cinnamon-and-diabetes
4. https://www.superfood-world.com/blogs/news/the-remarkable-anti-diabetic-effects-of-ceylon-cinnamon
5. https://diabetesjournals.org/care/article/30/9/2236/29314/Effect-of-Cinnamon-on-Glucose-and-Lipid-Levels-in
6. https://diabetesjournals.org/care/article/26/12/3215/21858/Cinnamon-Improves-Glucose-and-Lipids-of-People
7. https://dmsjournal.biomedcentral.com/articles/10.1186/s13098-023-01057

Chinese peony

1. Frontiers | Efficacy, Chemical Constituents, and Pharmacological Actions of Radix Paeoniae Rubra and Radix Paeoniae Alba
2. Does the extract of white peony root have benefits for diabetes? Are these all safe and applicable for diabetic patients?
3. Comprehensive chemical and bioactive investigation of Chinese peony flower
4. 10 medicinal constituents of Paeonia lactiflora (chinese peony)
5. 10 Best Active Constituents of Paeonia lactiflora (White Peony)
6. Sjögren's Symptoms Eased with Chinese Peony Compound, Trial Shows
7. A comprehensive review on traditional uses, phytochemistry and pharmacological properties of Paeonia emodi Wall. ex Royle

Chinese Yam

1. Diabetes Meal Plans. (n.d.). Yams and Diabetes. Retrieved from https://diabetesmealplans.com/17532/yams-and-diabetes/
2. SelfDecode Supplements. (2023). 6 Chinese Yam (Nagaimo) Benefits \u002B Nutrition \u0026 Side Effects. Retrieved from https://supplements.selfdecode.com/blog/chinese-yam/
3. Cambridge University Press. (2023). Could consumption of yam (Dioscorea) or its extract be beneficial in controlling glycaemia?. Retrieved from https://www.cambridge.org/core/journals/british-journal-of-nutrition/article/could-consumption-of-yam-dioscorea-or-its-extract-be-beneficial-in-controlling-glycaemia-a-systematic-review/42A0CF1169BA5A6F85F80E7950B35C43
4. JScholar Online. (2024). Research progress on the Active Ingredients and Pharmacological Effects of Yam. Retrieved from https://www.jscholaronline.org/articles/JACS/Active-Ingredients-and-Pharmacological-Effects-of-Yam.pdf
5. MDPI. (2023). Chinese Yam and Its Active Components Regulate the Structure of Gut Microbiota and Indole-like Metabolites in Anaerobic Fermentation In Vitro. Retrieved from https://www.mdpi.com/2072-6643/15/24/5112
6. MDPI. (2024). A Frontier Review of Nutraceutical Chinese Yam. Retrieved from https://www.mdpi.com/2304-8158/13/10/1426
7. MDPI. (2023). Dioscorea spp.: Bioactive Compounds and Potential for the Treatment of Inflammatory and Metabolic Diseases. Retrieved from https://www.mdpi.com/1420-3049/28/6/2878

Chromium

1. https://www.preventivemedicinedaily.com/diseases-conditions/endocrine/diabetes/chromium-and-vanadium-for-diabetes-benefits-and-research-findings/
2. https://link.springer.com/referenceworkentry/10.1007/978-1-4614-1533-6_20
3. https://www.diabetes.co.uk/Diabetes-and-Chromium.html
4. https://diabetesjournals.org/care/article/27/11/2741/23769/Role-of-Chromium-in-Human-Health-and-in-Diabetes
5. https://www.verywellhealth.com/chromium-benefits-4588421
6. https://academic.oup.com/nutritionreviews/article/74/7/455/1752210
7. https://diabetesjournals.org/diabetes/article/46/11/1786/10196/Elevated-Intakes-of-Supplemental-Chromium-Improve
8. https://www.researchsquare.com/article/rs-4059871/v1
9. https://ods.od.nih.gov/factsheets/Chromium-HealthProfessional/?adb_sid=e56947ea-97c5-4403-8bd6-aa7def393061
10. https://en.m.wikipedia.org/wiki/Chromium

Chrysanthemum

1. WebMD - Chrysanthemum: Uses, Side Effects, and More
2. WebMD - Health Benefits of Chrysanthemum Tea
3. RxList - Chrysanthemum: Health Benefits, Side Effects, Uses, Dose & Precautions
4. Biotech Asia - An Up-To-Date Review of Phytochemicals and Biological Activities in Chrysanthemum Spp
5. Chinese Medicine Research Hub - Chrysanthemum indicum L.: A Comprehensive Review of its Botany, Phytochemistry and Pharmacology

Copper

1. https://www.mdpi.com/2218-1989/13/1/17
2. https://link.springer.com/article/10.1007/s12011-016-0877-y
3. https://www.mdpi.com/2072-6643/15/7/1655
4. https://www.frontiersin.org/journals/public-health/articles/10.3389/fpubh.2024.1401347/full
5. https://www.mdpi.com/2072-6643/15/7/1655
6. https://diabetesjournals.org/diabetes/article/67/Supplement_1/1598-P/54229/Copper-Is-Associated-with-Metabolic-Syndrome-and

Creatine

1. https://www.mdpi.com/2072-6643/13/2/570
2. https://link.springer.com/article/10.1007/s00726-016-2277-1
3. https://observatorio.fm.usp.br/bitstream/OPI/39714/1/art_SOLIS_Potential_of_Creatine_in_Glucose_Management_and_Diabetes_2021.PDF
4. https://supplementsalon.com/creatine-and-diabetes/

Dandelion

1. https://www.medicalnewstoday.com/articles/324083
2. https://discover.texasrealfood.com/diabetes-diet-decoder/dandelion-greens
3. https://www.mountsinai.org/health-library/herb/dandelion
4. https://www.verywellhealth.com/the-benefits-of-dandelion-root-89103
5. https://www.healthline.com/nutrition/dandelion-benefits

Echinacea

1. https://www.healthline.com/nutrition/echinacea
2. https://feelgoodpal.com/blog/echinacea/
3. https://www.foodsforbetterhealth.com/is-echinacea-tea-healthy-benefits-and-side-effects-38090
4. https://www.verywellhealth.com/echinacea-benefits-side-effects-and-more-7503379
5. https://diabetesjournals.org/care/article/26/4/1277/23631/Systematic-Review-of-Herbs-and-Dietary-Supplements
6. https://www.nccih.nih.gov/health/echinacea
7. https://pmc.ncbi.nlm.nih.gov/articles/PMC3468018/

Fenugreek

1. Almatroodi, S. A., Almatroudi, A., Alsahli, M. A., & Rahmani, A. H. (2021). Fenugreek (Trigonella Foenum-Graecum) and its Active Compounds: A Review of its Effects on Human Health through Modulating Biological Activities. Pharmacognosy Journal, 13(3), 813-821.
2. Diabetes.co.uk. (2019). Fenugreek - Blood Sugar Levels Effects & Metabolism.

3. Healthline. (n.d.). How Fenugreek Can Help Control Blood Sugar.
4. Medical News Today. (n.d.). Fenugreek and diabetes: Links, benefits, and risks.
5. International Journal of Health & Medical Research. (2024). Active Ingredients and Antidiabetic Activity of Fenugreek: A Review Article.

Ginger

1. Healthline: Ginger and Diabetes
2. Medical News Today: Ginger for Diabetes
3. Everyday Health: Ginger and Diabetes
4. MDPI: Ginger Bioactives
5. Phytojournal: Ginger Chemical Constituents
6. Frontiers: Ginger Anti-inflammatory Actions
7. Frontiers: Ginger Antioxidant Mechanism

Ginkgo Biloba

1. DrugBank Online. "Ginkgo biloba: Uses, Interactions, Mechanism of Action." DrugBank, 2023.
2. Frontiers in Endocrinology. "Effects and safety of Ginkgo biloba on blood metabolism in type 2 diabetes mellitus: a systematic review and meta-analysis." 2023.
3. ScienceDaily. "Ginkgo biloba may aid in treating type 2 diabetes." 2019.
4. Neuroscience News. "Ginkgo biloba may aid in treating Type 2 Diabetes." 2019.
5. Molecules. "The Potential of Ginkgo biloba as a Source of Biologically Active Compounds." 2023.
6. Clinical Pharmacokinetics. "Ginkgo biloba Extracts: A Review of the Pharmacokinetics of the Active Ingredients." 2013.

Goji Berries

1. WebMD: Goji Berries: Health Benefits and Side Effects
2. TheHealthSite: Are Goji Berries Good For Diabetics? Explains Dietician
3. Medical News Today: 7 Goji Berry Benefits Backed by Science
4. Onlymyhealth: Are Goji Berries Good for Diabetics? Know from Experts
5. MDPI: Antitumor Mechanisms of Lycium barbarum Fruit: An Overview of In Vitro and In Vivo Potential

6. Wiley Online Library: Goji Berries as a Potential Natural Antioxidant Medicine: An Insight into Their Molecular Mechanisms of Action

Green Tea

1. https://www.medicalnewstoday.com/articles/tea-and-diabetes-2
2. https://www.eatingwell.com/article/7991760/green-tea-blood-sugar-gut-inflammation-new-study/
3. https://www.signos.com/blog/is-green-tea-good-for-type-2-diabetes
4. https://www.healthline.com/health/diabetes/green-tea-and-diabetes
5. https://nutritionandmetabolism.biomedcentral.com/articles/10.1186/s12986-020-00469-5
6. https://www.eatingwell.com/is-green-tea-good-for-you-8363574
7. https://nutritionandmetabolism.biomedcentral.com/counter/pdf/10.1186/s12986-020-00469-5.pdf
8. https://nutritionj.biomedcentral.com/articles/10.1186/1475-2891-9-63
9. https://academic.oup.com/nutritionreviews/advance-article-abstract/doi/10.1093/nutrit/nuae068/7696007

Gymnema-sylvestre

1. https://diabetesjournals.org/spectrum/article/22/4/206/2405/Dietary-Supplements-for-Diabetes-An-Evaluation-of
2. https://link.springer.com/chapter/10.1007/978-3-031-44914-7_8
3. https://supplements.selfdecode.com/blog/gymnema-sylvestre/
4. https://restorativemedicine.org/library/monographs/gymnema/
5. https://examine.com/supplements/gymnema-sylvestre

Hawthorn

1. Ulbricht, C., Basch, E., Cheung, L., et al. (2008). An evidence-based systematic review of hawthorn (Crataegus spp.) by the Natural Standard Research Collaboration. Journal of Dietary Supplements, 5(1), 63–94. **Taylor & Francis Online**
2. Walker, A. F., Marakis, G., Simpson, E., Hope, J. L. (2006). Hypotensive effects of hawthorn for patients with diabetes taking prescription drugs: a randomized controlled trial. British Journal of General Practice, 56(527), 437–443. **BJGP**
3. Chang, Q., Zuo, Z., Harrison, F., Chow, M. S. (2002). Hawthorn. Journal of Clinical Pharmacology, 42(6), 605–612. **SAGE Journals**
4. Liu, P., Kallio, H., Yang, B. (2011). Phenolic compounds in hawthorn (Crataegus grayana) fruits and leaves and changes during fruit

ripening. Journal of Agricultural and Food Chemistry, 59(20), 11141–11149. **ACS Publications**

5. Koch, E., Malek, F. A. (2011). Standardized extracts from hawthorn leaves and flowers (Crataegus spp.) with a defined content of oligomeric procyanidins. Wiener Medizinische Wochenschrift, 161(3-4), 65–72. **Springer Link**

6. Chang, W. C., Jia, H., Kuo, C. H., Chao, K., Cheng, T. H. (2005). Role of oxidative stress and defective insulin signaling in cardiovascular disorders. Biochemical and Biophysical Research Communications, 334(2), 449–456. **ScienceDirect**

7. National Center for Complementary and Integrative Health (NCCIH). (2020). Hawthorn. **NCCIH**

8. Peng, W., Wu, J. G., Jiang, Y. B., Liu, Y. J., Sun, T., Wu, N., Chen, S. W., Wu, C. J. (2015). Antidiabetic effects of hawthorn leaves flavonoids and epicatechin on diabetic rats induced by high-fat diet and streptozotocin. Food and Chemical Toxicology, 80, 231–239. **ScienceDirec**

Hydrangea

1. https://www.medicinenet.com/hydrangea_root_good_for_benefits_side_effects/article.htm
2. https://www.webmd.com/vitamins/ai/ingredientmono-663/hydrangea
3. https://facty.com/lifestyle/wellness/10-benefits-and-uses-of-hydrangeas/

Jujube

1. Scientific Origin: Is Eating Jujube Safe for People with Diabetes?
2. Health: Jujube (Chinese Red Date): Health Benefits and Risks
3. MDPI: A Literature Review of the Pharmacological Effects of Jujube
4. ResearchGate: A Literature Review of the Pharmacological Effects of Jujube
5. Verywell Health: What to Know About Eating Jujube Fruit (Chinese Dates)
6. Frontiers: A Review of Edible Jujube, the Ziziphus jujuba Fruit: A Heath Food Supplement for Anemia Prevalence
7. International Society for Horticultural Science: Biologically Active Components and Health Benefits of Jujube

Korean ginseng

1. https://www.medicalnewstoday.com/articles/ginseng-and-diabetes-type-2

2. https://www.herbazest.com/herbs/ginseng/ginseng-for-diabetes
3. https://centreforhealthyaging.org/physical-health/red-ginseng-for-diabetes-how-the-herb-stops-blood-sugar-from-spiking/
4. https://koreascience.kr/article/JAKO202010163510162.page

Lemon Balm

1. Anti-diabetic effects of lemon balm (Melissa officinalis) essential oil on glucose- and lipid-regulating enzymes in type 2 diabetic mice
2. Lemon Balm: Benefits, Side Effects, Dosage - Verywell Health
3. Lemon Balm Uses, Benefits, Side Effects and More - Dr. Axe
4. 7 Benefits of Lemon Balm \u002B Side Effects - SelfDecode Supplements
5. Health Benefits of Lemon Balm – WebMD

Leucine

1. Chen, Q., et al. (2018). Effects of Leucine Supplementation on Glycemic Control in Rodent Models of Type 2 Diabetes Mellitus: A Systematic Review and Meta-Analysis. Nutrients, 10(4), 585. https://www.mdpi.com/2072-6643/10/4/585
2. Zhang, Y., et al. (2007). Leucine Supplementation Improves Insulin Signaling via the mTOR Pathway in Skeletal Muscle of Rats. Nutrition, 23(11-12), 845-852. https://www.sciencedirect.com/science/article/pii/S0899900070700284 3
3. Yang, J., et al. (2010). Branched-Chain Amino Acid Supplementation Correlates with Improvement in Insulin Resistance Markers: A Meta-Analysis. Nutrition Journal, 9, 11. https://nutritionj.biomedcentral.com/articles/10.1186/1475-2891-9-11
4. Layman, D. K., et al. (2003). A Reduced Ratio of Dietary Carbohydrate to Protein Improves Body Composition and Blood Lipid Profiles during Weight Loss in Adult Women. Journal of Nutrition, 133(2), 411-417. https://academic.oup.com/jn/article/133/2/411/4818117
5. Newsholme, P., et al. (2005). Leucine and Glutamine Influence Cell Signaling and Insulin Secretion in Pancreatic Beta-Cells. Advances in Enzyme Regulation, 45, 209-226. https://www.sciencedirect.com/science/article/pii/S0065257105000015 8
6. Pedroso, F. E., et al. (2015). Leucine Supplementation Improves Insulin Sensitivity via mTORC2 Activation and Reverses Hepatic Steatosis in Diabetic Mice. American Journal of Physiology-Endocrinology and Metabolism, 309(8), E763-E771. https://journals.physiology.org/doi/full/10.1152/ajpendo.00453.2014

Licorice Root

1. WebMD - Health Benefits of Licorice Root
2. Weekand - Does Licorice Root Raise Blood Glucose?
3. NDTV - Diabetes Management: Licorice Root
4. Healthline - Licorice Root: Benefits, Uses, Precautions, and Dosage
5. ResearchGate - Licorice: Comprehensive Review of Its Chemical Composition
6. MDPI - Glycyrrhiza glabra (Licorice): A Comprehensive Review
7. SpringerLink - Phytochemical Constituents and Pharmacological Effects of Licorice

Magnesium

1. https://www.preventivemedicinedaily.com/diseases-conditions/endocrine/diabetes/magnesium-for-diabetes/
2. https://www.healthline.com/nutrition/is-magnesium-good-for-my-blood-sugar-levels-if-i-have-diabetes
3. https://www.medcentral.com/endocrinology/diabetes/the-role-of-magnesium-in-diabetes
4. https://www.verywellhealth.com/magnesium-in-type-2-diabetes-5184455
5. https://diabetesjournals.org/care/article/34/9/2116/38612/Magnesium-Intake-and-Risk-of-Type-2-DiabetesMeta
6. https://diabetesjournals.org/care/article/37/2/419/29258/Higher-Magnesium-Intake-Reduces-Risk-of-Impaired
7. https://www.healthline.com/health/diabetes/magnesium-and-diabetes
8. https://www.mdpi.com/2072-6643/13/2/320

Milk Thistle

1. Life Extension: Milk Thistle Reduces Elevated Glucose
2. Rupa Health: A Deep Dive into Milk Thistle's Potential Impact on Type 2 Diabetes
3. Cleveland Clinic: Milk Thistle: 6 Potential Benefits
4. MDPI: Milk Thistle and Diabetes: A Comprehensive Review
5. WebMD: Health Benefits of Milk Thistle

Nattokinase

1. https://drjessesantiano.com/how-to-dose-nattokinase-bromelain-and-nac/

2. https://www.webmd.com/diet/health-benefits-nattokinase
3. https://www.verywellhealth.com/what-is-nattokinase-89831
4. https://academic.oup.com/jes/article/4/Supplement_1/SAT-618/5834226
5. https://www.webmd.com/diet/health-benefits-nattokinase
6. https://cen.acs.org/acs-news/acs-meeting-news/Natto-fermented-soy-dish-controls/99/web/2021/08.
7. https://www.imrpress.com/journal/RCM/24/8/10.31083/j.rcm2408234/htm

Nitrosigine

1. https://www.frontiersin.org/journals/endocrinology/articles/10.3389/fendo.2023.1265372/full
2. https://diabetesjournals.org/compendia/article/2022/1/1/147001/Diagnosis-and-Treatment-of-Painful-Diabetic
3. https://diabetesjournals.org/care/article/36/9/2456/37875/Mechanisms-and-Management-of-Diabetic-Painful

NO3-T

1. https://supplements.selfdecode.com/blog/creatine-nitrate/
2. https://link.springer.com/article/10.1007/s00726-016-2277-1
3. https://cellucor.com/blogs/nutrition/creatine-nitrate
4. https://www.mdpi.com/2072-6643/13/2/5

Plantain

1. https://www.herbrally.com/monographs/plantain
2. https://www.researchgate.net/profile/Milad-Moloudizargari/publication/256494446_Therapeutic_Uses_and_Pharmacological_Properties_of_Plantago_major_L_and_its_Active_Constituents/links/02e7e5231a08c2fed3000000/Therapeutic-Uses-and-Pharmacological-Properties-of-Plantago-major-L-and-its-Active-Constituents.pdf
3. https://www.mdpi.com/1424-8247/16/8/1092
4. https://bmccomplementmedtherapies.biomedcentral.com/articles/10.1186/s12906-024-04621-z
5. https://auctoresonline.org/article/pharmacological-and-biochemical-activities-of-plantago-major

Poria

1. Chang, W., Chen, L., Hatch, G. M. (2015). Effect of Poria cocos polysaccharides on streptozotocin-induced diabetic symptoms in mice. Journal of Ethnopharmacology, 169, 22-30. **ScienceDirect**
2. Zhao, Y., Bleakley, B., Changalov, M. (2014). A review of the pharmacology and clinical effects of Poria cocos. Mushroom Research, 23(2), 8-13.
3. Zhang, H., Liu, M., Zhang, Y. (2019). Polysaccharides from Poria cocos attenuate hyperglycemia and hyperlipidemia in alloxan-induced diabetic mice. International Journal of Biological Macromolecules, 133, 320-328. **NCBI**
4. Xu, T., Beelman, R. B., Lambert, J. D. (2012). The cancer preventive effects of edible mushrooms. Anti-Cancer Agents in Medicinal Chemistry, 12(10), 1255-1263. **Bentham Science**
5. Shen, N., Wang, T., Gan, Q., Liu, S., Wang, L. (2012). The anti-diabetic activity of triterpenoids-rich extracts from Poria cocos. Journal of Medicinal Plants Research, 6(9), 1733-1739. **Academic Journals**
6. Chinese Pharmacopoeia Commission. (2015). Pharmacopoeia of the People's Republic of China. China Medical Science Press.
7. Cheung, F. (2011). TCM: Made in China. Nature, 480(7378), S82-S83.

Psyllium Husk

1. https://diabetesmealplans.com/12476/psyllium-husk-for-diabetes/
2. https://health.clevelandclinic.org/psyllium-husk
3. https://www.medicalnewstoday.com/articles/318707
4. https://www.wellnessverge.com/psyllium-husk-benefits-dosage-side-effects-sources

Raspberry extract

1. https://medicalxpress.com/news/2019-02-red-raspberries-glucose-people-pre-diabetes.html
2. https://discover.texasrealfood.com/diabetes-diet-decoder/raspberries
3. https://diabetesmealplans.com/11211/raspberries-and-type-2-diabetes/
4. https://www.mdpi.com/1660-4601/18/17/9364
5. https://diabetesmealplans.com/11211/raspberries-and-type-2-diabetes/
6. https://www.researchgate.net/profile/Angelos-Sikalidis/publication/354362587_Effects_of_Dietary_Red_Raspberry_Consumption_on_Pre-Diabetes_and_Type_2_Diabetes_Mellitus_Parameters/links/61337e8

5c69a4e48797cf922/Effects-of-Dietary-Red-Raspberry-Consumption-on-Pre-Diabetes-and-Type-2-Diabetes-Mellitus-Parameters.pdf
7. https://www.academia.edu/51914388/Effects_of_Dietary_Red_Raspb
    erry_Consumption_on_Pre_Diabetes_and_Type_2_Diabetes_Mellitus
    _Parameters

Rehmannia

1. Dr. Axe. "Rehmannia Root Benefits, Uses, Side Effects and More." Dr. Axe, 7 Oct. 2018, https://draxe.com/nutrition/rehmannia/.
2. WebMD. "Rehmannia: Uses, Side Effects, and More." WebMD, https://www.webmd.com/vitamins/ai/ingredientmono-1155/rehmannia.
3. RxList. "Rehmannia: Health Benefits, Side Effects, Uses, Dose & Precautions." RxList, https://www.rxlist.com/supplements/rehmannia.htm.

Resveratrol

1. https://diabetesmealplans.com/15832/resveratrol-for-diabetes/
2. https://naomiw.com/blogs/nutrition/resveratrol-and-high-blood-sugar-keep-your-levels-healthy
3. https://link.springer.com/article/10.1007/s11033-023-08746-1
4. https://diabetesjournals.org/care/article/39/12/2211/31874/Resveratrol-as-Add-on-Therapy-in-Subjects-With
5. https://www.healthline.com/health-news/resveratrol-beneficial-for-diabetes
6. https://ajcn.nutrition.org/

Schisandra

1. WebMD: Schisandra Uses and Risks
2. MediChannel: Schisandra for Diabetes
3. Dr. Axe: Schisandra Benefits, Uses, Forms and Side Effects
4. Frontiers in Nutrition: Nutritional Effects of Schisandra chinensis
5. Rainwood Bio: Active Ingredients of Schisandra Extract
6. Memorial Sloan Kettering Cancer Center: Schisandra
7. Human Clinical Studies: Schisandra

Sumac

1. https://www.mdpi.com/2076-3921/10/1/73
2. https://link.springer.com/article/10.1007/s11694-019-00077-9

3. https://link.springer.com/article/10.1007/s11892-018-1042-0
4. https://www.mdpi.com/2311-7524/8/12/1168
5. https://www.frontiersin.org/journals/nutrition/articles/10.3389/fnut.2024.1305024/full

THC Marijuana

1. https://www.verywellhealth.com/marijuana-and-diabetes-5105170
2. https://www.diabetesdaily.com/learn-about-diabetes/living-with-diabetes/diabetes-and-work-life-play/marijuana-and-diabetes-what-you-need-to-know/
3. https://www.diabetescarecommunity.ca/living-well-with-diabetes-articles/what-you-should-know-about-diabetes-and-recreational-marijuana/
4. https://www.diabetescarecommunity.ca/living-well-with-diabetes-articles/what-you-should-know-about-diabetes-and-recreational-marijuana/

Turmeric

1. https://www.healthline.com/health/diabetes/turmeric-and-diabetes
2. https://www.verywellhealth.com/turmeric-effect-on-diabetes-5120109
3. https://www.everydayhealth.com/type-2-diabetes/can-turmeric-help-prevent-treat-diabetes/
4. https://www.frontiersin.org/journals/endocrinology/articles/10.3389/fendo.2021.669448/full
5. https://pmc.ncbi.nlm.nih.gov/articles/PMC3288651/
6. https://www.sugarfit.com/blog/benefits-of-turmeric-for-diabetes/
7. https://pubs.rsc.org/en/content/articlelanding/2022/fo/d2fo02625b
8. https://link.springer.com/article/10.1007/s11010-021-04201-6
9. https://link.springer.com/chapter/10.1007/978-3-030-56153-6_8

Vanadium

1. https://www.preventivemedicinedaily.com/diseases-conditions/endocrine/diabetes/chromium-and-vanadium-for-diabetes-benefits-and-research-findings/
2. https://www.mountsinai.org/health-library/supplement/vanadium
3. https://supplementsinreview.com/blood-sugar/vanadium-blood-sugar/

4. https://diabetesjournals.org/spectrum/article/22/4/214/2326/The-Role-of-Micronutrients-in-Managing-Diabetes
5. https://diabetesjournals.org/spectrum/article/14/3/133/654/Select-Vitamins-and-Minerals-in-the-Management-of
6. https://link.springer.com/content/pdf/10.1007/s12011-018-1540-6.pdf
7. https://link.springer.com/article/10.1023/A:1007067011338
8. https://www.mdpi.com/1422-0067/24/21/15675

Vitamin B8

1. Pacioni, D., et al. (2020). *Myo-inositol and its effects on insulin resistance and metabolic diseases: A summary of current evidence.* Journal of Nutritional Science, 9, e20. Link
2. D'Anna, R., et al. (2017). *Myo-inositol and D-chiro-inositol supplementation in overweight pregnant women with gestational diabetes mellitus: Effects on metabolic profile and pregnancy outcomes.* European Review for Medical and Pharmacological Sciences, 21(22), 5011-5020. Link
3. Laganà, A. S., et al. (2018). *Inositol and polycystic ovary syndrome: From pathogenesis to treatment.* Gynecological Endocrinology, 34(7), 512-517. Link
4. Croze, M. L., & Soulage, C. O. (2013). *Potential role and therapeutic interests of myo-inositol in metabolic diseases.* Biochimie, 95(10), 1811-1827. Link
5. Genazzani, A. D., et al. (2016). *Effects of a combination of myo-inositol and D-chiro-inositol on metabolic and hormonal parameters in women with polycystic ovary syndrome (PCOS).* Gynecological Endocrinology, 32(1), 69-73. Link
6. Unfer, V., et al. (2017). *Effects of myo-inositol in women with gestational diabetes: A randomized controlled trial.* Journal of Maternal-Fetal & Neonatal Medicine, 30(17), 2166-2169. Link

Vitamin D3

1. Verywell Health - Vitamin D and Type 2 Diabetes
2. Medical News Today - Diabetes and Vitamin D
3. Healthline - Vitamin D2 vs. D3
4. Diabetes.co.uk - Vitamin D and Diabetes
5. American Diabetes Association - Vitamin D & Insulin Resistance

White Mulberry

1. WebMD - White Mulberry
2. Diabetes Daily - Does White Mulberry Leaf Help Diabetes?
3. Verywell Health - White Mulberry Benefits and Side Effects
4. MDPI - Biosynthesis and Pharmacological Activities of the Bioactive Compounds of White Mulberry
5. Frontiers in Pharmacology - Novel active compounds and the anti-diabetic mechanism of mulberry leaves
6. Drugs.com - White Mulberry Uses, Benefits & Dosage

Wormwood

1. https://ediblealaska.ediblecommunities.com/food-thought/wormwood-its-history-and-use
2. https://www.medicalnewstoday.com/articles/wormwood
3. https://yalebooks.yale.edu/2020/08/14/diabetes-among-native-americans/
4. https://diabetesjournals.org/spectrum/article/23/4/272/31851/Traditions-and-Diabetes-Prevention-A-Healthy-Path
5. https://broadview.org/the-link-between-diabetes-among-indigenous-peoples-and-colonialism/
6. https://diabetesjournals.org/spectrum/article/23/4/272/31851/Traditions-and-Diabetes-Prevention-A-Healthy-Path
7. https://diabetesfoodhub.org/blog/what-are-natural-sugars-and-how-do-they-impact-diabetes
8. https://botanicalinstitute.org/artemisia-annua/
9. https://www.utep.edu/herbal-safety/herbal-facts/herbal%20facts%20sheet/wormwood.html
10. https://en.m.wikipedia.org/wiki/Artemisia_absinthium
11. https://www.ancientherbswisdom.com/wormwood-50-questions-and-answers/
12. https://www.fs.usda.gov/database/feis/plants/forb/artabs/all.html

Neuropathy

Contents

Neuropathy and its connections to diabetes

1. Chen, Y., Sun, L., Chen, M., Zhang, H., Song, B., Wang, H., Jiang, A., Zhang, L., Li, S., Wang, J., & Wang, W. (2024). Lower Free Triiodothyronine is a Risk Factor of Diabetic Peripheral Neuropathy in Patients with Type 2 Diabetes Mellitus. Diabetes Metab Syndr Obes, 17:4407-4415.
2. Cleveland Clinic. (n.d.). Diabetes-Related Neuropathy: What It Is, Symptoms & Treatment. Retrieved from Cleveland Clinic.
3. Mayo Clinic. (n.d.). Diabetic Neuropathy - Symptoms & Causes. Retrieved from Mayo Clinic.
4. American Diabetes Association. (n.d.). Understanding Neuropathy and Your Diabetes. Retrieved from American Diabetes Association.
5. Healthline. (2024). How Long Do You Have Diabetes Before Neuropathy?. Retrieved from Healthline.

The Myelin Sheath

1. https://my.clevelandclinic.org/health/body/22974-myelin-sheath
2. https://www.verywellhealth.com/myelin-sheath-4129059
3. https://medlineplus.gov/ency/article/002261.htm
4. https://www.elsevier.com/resources/anatomy/cells-of-nervous-tissue/myelin-sheath/myelin-sheath/15379

Acetyl L-Carnitine

1. https://link.springer.com/article/10.1007/s11064-023-03911-1
2. https://diabetesjournals.org/care/article/28/1/89/25830/Acetyl-l-Carnitine-Improves-Pain-Nerve
3. https://www.mdpi.com/2072-6643/12/5/1389
4. https://link.springer.com/article/10.2165/00023210-200721001-00005

Alpha Lipoic Acid

1. https://www.mdpi.com/2076-3921/13/10/1228
2. https://www.mdpi.com/2076-3921/11/12/2420
3. https://www.activeala.com/alpha-lipoic-acid-for-neuropathy/
4. https://www.mdpi.com/2072-6643/15/16/3634
5. https://examine.com/supplements/alpha-lipoic-acid/

Arnica

1. Leu, S., Havey, K. D., White, L. E., Martin, N., Yoo, S. S., & Rademaker, A. W. (2010). Accelerated resolution of laser-induced bruising with topical 20% arnica: a rater-blinded randomized controlled trial. *British Journal of Dermatology*, 163(3), 557-563. doi:10.1111/j.1365-2133.2010.09833.x
2. Kneusel, O., Muggli, R., & Suter, A. (2002). Arnica Montana gel in osteoarthritis of the knee: an open, multicenter clinical trial. *Advances in Therapy*, 19(5), 209-218. doi:10.1007/BF02850281
3. Memorial Sloan Kettering Cancer Center. (2021). Arnica. Retrieved from https://www.mskcc.org/cancer-care/integrative-medicine/herbs/arnica
4. Cleveland Clinic. (2020). Arnica: What It Is and How To Use It. Retrieved from https://health.clevelandclinic.org/arnica-should-you-use-it/
5. Calgary Neuropathy Association. (n.d.). Arnica – A Natural Solution to Neuropathy Symptoms. Retrieved from https://calgaryneuropathy.com/arnica-natural-solution-neuropathy-symptoms/
6. Mills, S., & Bone, K. (2013). *Principles and Practice of Phytotherapy: Modern Herbal Medicine* (2nd ed.). Churchill Livingstone Elsevier.
7. Newall, C. A., Anderson, L. A., & Phillipson, J. D. (1996). *Herbal Medicines: A Guide for Health-Care Professionals*. Pharmaceutical Press.
8. Natural Medicines Comprehensive Database. (2021). Arnica. Retrieved from https://naturalmedicines.therapeuticresearch.com

Bearberry

1. MedicineNet. "Bearberry: UTI Uses, Benefits, Side Effects, Warnings." MedicineNet
2. WholisticMatters. "Bearberry (Uva Ursi) Benefits for Urinary Health & More." WholisticMatters
3. Beauty Setup. "Bearberry | Beauty Setup." Beauty Setup
4. Herbal Supplement Resource. "Bearberry - Side Effects, Uses and Benefits." Herbal Supplement Resource

Benfotiamine

1. https://lifetreehq.com/benfotiamine-for-neuropathy/

2. https://www.longlifenutri.com/blogs/news/can-benfotiamine-reverse-the-neuropathy
3. https://www.alzdiscovery.org/uploads/cognitive_vitality_media/Benfotiamine-Cognitive-Vitality-For-Researchers.pdf
4. https://www.mdpi.com/1422-0067/22/11/5418
5. https://europeanreview.org/wp/wp-content/uploads/3261-3273.pdf
6. https://en.m.wikipedia.org/wiki/Benfotiamine

Bitterroot

1. Anand, P., & Katz, R. (2010). Management of chronic neuropathic pain: the need for "top down" rather than "bottom up" therapeutics. *The FASEB Journal*, 24(12), 4564-4570. https://doi.org/10.1096/fj.10-163816
2. Chevallier, A. (1996). *The Encyclopedia of Medicinal Plants*. DK Publishing.
3. Elsas, S. M., Rossi, D. J., Raber, J., White, G., Seeley, C. A., Gregory, W. L., ... & Soumyanath, A. (2010). Extracts of *Withania somnifera* root and purified *withanolides* protect against glutamate excitotoxicity. *Phytotherapy Research*, 24(7), 948-954. https://doi.org/10.1002/ptr.3024
4. Hart, J. A. (1976). Montana native plants and early peoples. *Montana Historical Society Press*.
5. Krochmal, A., Walters, R. S., & Doughty, R. M. (1960). A guide to medicinal plants of Appalachia. *USDA Forest Service Agriculture Handbook*, No. 400.
6. Moerman, D. E. (1998). *Native American Ethnobotany*. Timber Press.
7. Sas, K., Robotka, H., Toldi, J., & Vécsei, L. (2018). Mitochondria, oxidative stress and the kynurenine system, with a focus on neurodegenerative disorders. *Journal of the Neurological Sciences*, 368, 196-206. https://doi.org/10.1016/j.jns.2016.10.018
8. Turner, N. J., Bouchard, R., & Kennedy, D. I. D. (1980). *Ethnobotany of the Okanagan-Colville Indians of British Columbia and Washington*. British Columbia Provincial Museum.

BPC-157

1. https://www.cochrane-handbook.org/bpc-157-tablets-vs-injection-weighing-the-pros-and-cons/
2. https://www.predatornutrition.com/articlesdetail?cid=bpc-157-benefits-and-side-effects
3. https://propeptidesource.com/the-potential-of-bpc-157-in-treating-neurological-conditions-a-comprehensive-review/

4. https://mentalhealthdaily.com/2024/01/02/bpc-157-peptide-for-neurological-cns-disorders-preliminary-research/

Chinese Peony

1. He, D.-Y., & Dai, S.-M. (2011). Anti-inflammatory and immunomodulatory effects of Paeonia lactiflora Pall., a traditional Chinese herbal medicine. Frontiers in Pharmacology, 2, 10. **Frontiers in Pharmacology**
2. Wang, D., Sun, H., Song, G., & Li, L. (2018). Paeoniflorin attenuates diabetic peripheral neuropathy through inflammation suppression in streptozotocin-induced diabetic rats. Acta Cirúrgica Brasileira, 33(8), 676–683. **Acta Cirúrgica Brasileira**
3. Zhang, H., Li, S., Zhang, D., Wang, Y., & Zhao, L. (2019). Paeoniflorin ameliorates neuropathic pain by regulating TLR4/MyD88/NF-κB signaling pathway. Pharmaceutical Biology, 57(1), 778–784. **Pharmaceutical Biology**
4. Shen, Y., Li, C. G., Zhou, S. F., Pang, E. C., Story, D. F., & Xue, C. C. (2008). Paeonia lactiflora extract inhibits production of nitric oxide and proinflammatory cytokines in stimulated human monocytic cells. Journal of Ethnopharmacology, 119(2), 343–350. **Journal of Ethnopharmacology**
5. Chinese Pharmacopoeia Commission. (2015). Pharmacopoeia of the People's Republic of China. Beijing: China Medical Science Press.
6. Kim, J. H., Jeong, K. S., & Kim, G. Y. (2010). Anti-inflammatory effects of Paeonia lactiflora on carrageenan-induced paw edema in rats. Journal of Ethnopharmacology, 128(2), 221–226. **Journal of Ethnopharmacology**
7. Li, J., Zhao, Y., & Si, X. (2017). Protective effect of paeoniflorin against chemotherapy-induced peripheral neuropathy in mice through inhibition of oxidative stress and neuroinflammation. Biomedicine & Pharmacotherapy, 95, 904–910. **Biomedicine & Pharmacotherapy**

Chrysanthemum

1. Chen, R., Qi, Q. L., Wang, M. T., & Li, Q. Y. (2010). Therapeutic potential of Chrysanthemum indicum Linn. in diseases. Molecules, 15(3), 1873–1886. MDPI
2. **Butt, M. S., Sultan, M. T., Aziz, M. (2009). Nutritional Profile of Chrysanthemum morifolium Flowers and Their Health Benefits. Journal of Medicinal Plants Research, 3(12), 815–820. Academic Journals
3. Ali, A., Wu, H., & Xie, N. (2018). Anti-inflammatory and antiviral effects of Chrysanthemum indicum Linnaeus, a Chinese medicinal herb, in vitro and in vivo. Journal of Ethnopharmacology, 220, 123–130. ScienceDirect

4. **He, C. N., Wang, C. L., Guo, S. X., & Yang, J. S. (2012). Research Progress on Chemical Constituents of Chrysanthemum morifolium Ramat and Their Pharmacological Activities. Chinese Herbal Medicines, 4(3), 178–188. ScienceDirect

5. Yang, Y., Yan, S., & Zhang, L. (2015). Neuroprotective Effect of Luteolin Against Chronic Cerebral Hypoperfusion-Induced Neurodegeneration Through Suppression of Neuroinflammation and Oxidative Stress. Neuroscience Letters, 585, 43–48. ScienceDirect

6. **Park, C. M., & Song, Y. S. (2013). Luteolin and Luteolin-7-O-glucoside Compounds Isolated from Chrysanthemum indicum Linne Prevent the Hepatic Fibrosis Induced by Thioacetamide in Rats. Journal of Ethnopharmacology, 146(2), choladecoder.com/97961479)

7. National Center for Complementary and Integrative Health. (2016). Herbs at a Glance: Chrysanthemum. NCCIH

Co-Q-10

1. https://link.springer.com/article/10.1007/s40495-021-00273-6

2. https://link.springer.com/article/10.1007/s00210-021-02161-8

3. https://pubs.asahq.org/anesthesiology/article/118/4/945/11324/Prophylactic-and-Antinociceptive-Effects-of

4. https://link.springer.com/article/10.1007/s00228-022-03407-x

5. https://link.springer.com/content/pdf/10.1007/s00228-022-03407-x.pdf

Curcumin

1. https://link.springer.com/article/10.1007/s10787-024-01492-1

2. https://link.springer.com/article/10.1007/s43440-020-00112-3

3. https://encyclopedia.pub/entry/2638

4. https://bmccomplementmedtherapies.biomedcentral.com/articles/10.1186/s12906-020-2867-z

Dandelion

1. Blumenthal, M., Goldberg, A., & Brinckmann, J. (Eds.). (2000). *Herbal Medicine: Expanded Commission E Monographs*. American Botanical Council.

2. Brinker, F. (2010). *Herbal Contraindications and Drug Interactions Plus Herbal Adjuncts with Medicines* (4th ed.). Eclectic Medical Publications.

3. Clare, B. A., Conroy, R. S., & Spelman, K. (2009). The diuretic effect in human subjects of an extract of Taraxacum officinale folium over a

single day. *Journal of Alternative and Complementary Medicine*, 15(8), 929-934. https://doi.org/10.1089/acm.2008.0152

4. Hu, C., & Kitts, D. D. (2005). Dandelion (Taraxacum officinale) flower extract suppresses both reactive oxygen species and nitric oxide and prevents lipid oxidation in vitro. *Phytomedicine*, 12(8), 588-597. https://doi.org/10.1016/j.phymed.2004.09.005

5. Martinez, M., Poirrier, P., Chamy, R., Leibovici, C., & Delmulle, L. (2015). Taraxacum officinale and related species – An ethnopharmacological review and its potential as a commercial medicinal plant. *Journal of Ethnopharmacology*, 169, 244-262. https://doi.org/10.1016/j.jep.2015.03.067

6. Schütz, K., Carle, R., & Schieber, A. (2006). Taraxacum—a review on its phytochemical and pharmacological profile. *Journal of Ethnopharmacology*, 107(3), 313-323. https://doi.org/10.1016/j.jep.2006.07.021

7. Natural Medicines Comprehensive Database. (2021). Dandelion. Retrieved from https://naturalmedicines.therapeuticresearch.com

8. University of Maryland Medical Center. (2015). Dandelion. Retrieved from https://www.umms.org/health/health-services/alternative-medicine/herb/dandelion

GABA

1. https://www.mdpi.com/1661-3821/4/2/15
2. https://www.sciencedaily.com/releases/2013/08/130805113430.htm
3. https://bmcrheumatol.biomedcentral.com/articles/10.1186/s41927-022-00257-z
4. https://link.springer.com/article/10.1007/s12272-013-0057-y
5. https://www.mdpi.com/1424-8247/17/5/623

Gamma Linolenic Acid

1. https://go.drugbank.com/drugs/DB13854
2. https://academic.oup.com/jn/article/137/2/368/4664546
3. https://nootropicology.com/alphalipoic-acid/

Ginko Biloba

1. Mahadevan, S., & Park, Y. (2008). Multifaceted therapeutic benefits of Ginkgo biloba L.: Chemistry, efficacy, safety, and uses. Journal of Food Science, 73(1), R14-R19. https://doi.org/10.1111/j.1750-3841.2007.00597.x
2. : Ahlemeyer, B., & Krieglstein, J. (2003). Neuroprotective effects of Ginkgo biloba extract. Cellular and Molecular Life Sciences, 60(9), 1779-1792. https://doi.org/10.1007/s00018-003-3086-7
3. : Tanaka, K., et al. (2004). Neuroprotective effects of bilobalide on energy deprivation-induced neuronal cell death in vitro. Journal of Neuroscience Research, 76(4), 453-459. https://doi.org/10.1002/jnr.20082
4. : Singh, B., & Srivastava, S. K. (2012). Anti-inflammatory and analgesic agents from Indian medicinal plants. International Journal of Integrative Biology, 13(1), 23-34.
5. : Maclennan, K. M., Darlington, C. L., & Smith, P. F. (2002). The CNS effects of Ginkgo biloba extracts and ginkgolide B. Progress in Neurobiology, 67(3), 235-257. https://doi.org/10.1016/S0301-0082(02)00010-8
6. : Kennedy, D. O., & Scholey, A. B. (2002). Ginkgo biloba: A potential neuroprotective agent in ischemia. Current Topics in Nutraceutical Research, 1(2), 121-136.
7. : Pittler, M. H., & Ernst, E. (2000). Ginkgo biloba extract for the treatment of intermittent claudication: A meta-analysis of randomized trials. The American Journal of Medicine, 108(4), 276-281. https://doi.org/10.1016/S0002-9343(99)00435-7

Hawthorn

1. Rigelsky, J. M., & Sweet, B. V. (2002). Hawthorn: Pharmacology and therapeutic uses. American Journal of Health-System Pharmacy, 59(5), 417–422. **American Journal of Health-System Pharmacy**
2. Chang, W., Dao, J., & Shao, Z. (2005). Neuroprotective effect of hawthorn extract in rat brain with transient focal ischemia. Journal of Ethnopharmacology, 101(1-3), 148–153. **Journal of Ethnopharmacology**
3. Bahorun, T., Gressier, B., Trotin, F., et al. (1996). Oxygen species scavenging activity of phenolic extracts from hawthorn fresh plant organs and pharmaceutical preparations. Arzneimittel-Forschung, 46(11), 1086–1089. **PubMed**
4. Koch, E., & Malek, F. A. (2011). Standardized extracts from hawthorn leaves and flowers (Crataegus spp.): Equivalence of clinical efficacy with differing oligomeric procyanidin content. Wiener Medizinische Wochenschrift, 161(3–4), 66–72. **SpringerLink**
5. Walker, A. F., Marakis, G., Simpson, E., Hope, J. L., Robinson, P. A., & Hassanein, M. (2006). Hypotensive effects of hawthorn for patients with diabetes taking prescription drugs: A randomized controlled trial.

British Journal of General Practice, 56(527), 437–443. **British Journal of General Practice**

6. Zhang, Z., & Ho, W. K. K. (2009). Neuroprotective effects of hawthorn extract on ischemia/reperfusion-induced cerebral injury. Brain Research, 1251, 204–212. **Brain Research**
7. Blumenthal, M., Goldberg, A., & Brinckmann, J. (Eds.). (2000). Herbal Medicine: Expanded Commission E Monographs. Austin, TX: American Botanical Council.

L-Arginine

1. https://l-arginine.com/l-arginine-and-neuropathy/
2. https://link.springer.com/article/10.1007/s10753-024-02139-7
3. https://www.frontiersin.org/journals/molecular-neuroscience/articles/10.3389/fnmol.2021.759729/full
4. https://link.springer.com/article/10.1007/s00394-017-1508-x
5. https://altmedrev.com/wp-content/uploads/2019/02/v11-4-294.pdf

L-Citrulline

1. https://www.webmd.com/vitamins-and-supplements/l-citrulline-uses-and-risks
2. https://www.verywellhealth.com/citrulline-4774848
3. https://health.clevelandclinic.org/citrulline-benefits
4. https://www.frontiersin.org/journals/pharmacology/articles/10.3389/fphar.2020.584669/full
5. https://www.mdpi.com/2076-3417/11/7/3293

Lions Mane

1. https://medshun.com/article/is-lion-mane-good-for-stroke-patients
2. https://tonikfusion.com/blogs/articles/can-lions-mane-help-nerve-damage
3. https://www.verywellfit.com/lion-s-mane-nutrition-facts-and-health-benefits-5185393
4. https://www.remeday.com/mushrooms/lions-mane-neuropathy
5. https://examine.com/supplements/lionsmane/

Magnesium

1. Abraham, G. E., & Flechas, J. D. (1992). Management of fibromyalgia: rationale for the use of magnesium and malic acid. *Journal of Nutritional Medicine*, 3(1), 49-59. https://doi.org/10.3109/13590849209003110

2. Altura, B. M., & Altura, B. T. (1984). Magnesium deficiency and cardiac arrhythmias. In *Magnesium in Health and Disease* (pp. 313-344). Spectrum Publications.

3. Bahgat, A., Abdel-Aziem, S. H., Helmy, H. S., & Anwer, K. (2016). Magnesium enhances the anti-inflammatory effect of gabapentin in a rat model of carrageenan-induced hind paw inflammation. *Clinical and Experimental Pharmacology and Physiology*, 43(12), 1164-1169. https://doi.org/10.1111/1440-1681.12645

4. Barbosa, K., Barchini, J., Bittencourt, L., & Paiva, A. (2012). Magnesium supplementation attenuates oxidative stress in streptozotocin-induced diabetic rats. *Journal of Diabetes & Metabolism*, 3(7), 1-5. https://doi.org/10.4172/2155-6156.1000216

5. Caddell, J. L. (1996). Magnesium and neural function: a hypothesis. *Magnesium Research*, 9(1), 65-77.

6. Freguin-Bouilland, C., Tison, F., & Debilly, B. (2013). Neuropathic pain improved with magnesium supplementation in a patient with prediabetes. *Journal of Pain and Symptom Management*, 45(2), e7-e9. https://doi.org/10.1016/j.jpainsymman.2012.07.012

7. Gröber, U., Schmidt, J., & Kisters, K. (2015). Magnesium in prevention and therapy. *Nutrients*, 7(9), 8199-8226. https://doi.org/10.3390/nu7095388

8. Iseri, L. T., & French, J. H. (1984). Magnesium: nature's physiologic calcium blocker. *American Heart Journal*, 108(1), 188-193. https://doi.org/10.1016/0002-8703(84)90550-5

9. Maier, J. A., Malpuech-Brugère, C., Zimowska, W., Rayssiguier, Y., & Mazur, A. (2004). Low magnesium promotes endothelial cell dysfunction: implications for atherosclerosis, inflammation and thrombosis. *Biochimica et Biophysica Acta (BBA) - Molecular Basis of Disease*, 1689(1), 13-21. https://doi.org/10.1016/j.bbadis.2004.01.002

10. National Institutes of Health, Office of Dietary Supplements. (2021). *Magnesium Fact Sheet for Health Professionals*. Retrieved from https://ods.od.nih.gov/factsheets/Magnesium-HealthProfessional/

11. Nielsen, F. H. (2010). Magnesium, inflammation, and obesity in chronic disease. *Nutrition Reviews*, 68(6), 333-340. https://doi.org/10.1111/j.1753-4887.2010.00293.x

12. Schuette, S. A., Lashner, B. A., & Janghorbani, M. (1994). Bioavailability of magnesium diglycinate vs magnesium oxide in patients with ileal resection. *JPEN. Journal of Parenteral and Enteral*

Nutrition, 18(5), 430-435.
https://doi.org/10.1177/0148607194018005430

13. Slutsky, I., Abumaria, N., Wu, L. J., Huang, C., Zhang, L., Li, B., ... & Liu, G. (2010). Enhancement of learning and memory by elevating brain magnesium. *Neuron*, 65(2), 165-177. https://doi.org/10.1016/j.neuron.2009.12.026

14. Song, Y., Li, T. Y., van Dam, R. M., & Hu, F. B. (2012). Magnesium intake and plasma concentrations in relation to systemic inflammation, insulin resistance, and the incidence of diabetes. *Diabetes Care*, 30(12), 3254–3260. https://doi.org/10.2337/dc07-1045

15. Walker, A. F., Marakis, G., Christie, S., Simpson, H. C. R., Byng, M., & Mg-OK Study Group. (2003). Mg citrate found more bioavailable than other Mg preparations in a randomised, double-blind study. *Magnesium Research*, 16(3), 183-191.

16. Weglicki, W. B., Chuang, S. T., Wu, X., Dhar, A., & Tepper, P. (1992). Role of magnesium deficiency in neuropathology. *Magnesium and Trace Elements*, 10(2-4), 105-113.

N-Acetyl L-Cysteine

1. https://europepmc.org/article/MED/24683506
2. https://onlinelibrary.wiley.com/doi/epdf/10.1002/brb3.208
3. https://www.mdpi.com/2076-3921/12/12/2073
4. https://link.springer.com/article/10.1080/14734220601142878
5. https://pmc.ncbi.nlm.nih.gov/articles/PMC8234027/

Omega 3 Fatty Acid

1. https://academic.oup.com/nutritionreviews/article/78/4/323/5571403
2. https://bmjopen.bmj.com/content/8/3/e020804
3. https://www.dovepress.com/effects-of-omega-3-polyunsaturated-fatty-acid-supplementation-on-neuro-peer-reviewed-fulltext-article-DMSO
4. https://www.sciencedaily.com/releases/2012/01/120111103856.htm
5. https://orcid.org/0000-0002-1596-2259

Peppermint

1. https://www.mdpi.com/1420-3049/28/9/3771
2. https://link.springer.com/article/10.1007/s11916-021-00959-y
3. https://www.jpsr.pharmainfo.in/Documents/Volumes/vol7Issue07/jpsr07071524.pdf

Plantain

1. Chiang, L. C., Chiang, W., Chang, M. Y., Ng, L. T., & Lin, C. C. (2002). Antiviral activity of Plantago major extracts and related compounds in vitro. *Antiviral Research*, 55(1), 53-62. https://doi.org/10.1016/S0166-3542(02)00006-3

2. Gálvez, M., Martín-Cordero, C., Houghton, P. J., & Ayuso, M. J. (2005). Antioxidant activity of methanol extracts obtained from Plantago species. *Journal of Agricultural and Food Chemistry*, 53(6), 1927-1933. https://doi.org/10.1021/jf040386v

3. Ji, K. M., Cheng, Z. Y., Zhang, S. Q., Chen, T. T., & Wang, Q. (2012). Anti-inflammatory and antioxidant properties of luteolin-7-O-beta-D-glucoside from Pyrola incarnata Fisch. leaves. *Fitoterapia*, 83(2), 323-330. https://doi.org/10.1016/j.fitote.2011.11.009

4. Paul, E. M., Ding, S., Ward, B. M., & Meyer, T. J. (2011). Immunomodulatory Activity of Plantago major Polysaccharides on Macrophage Functions. *International Journal of Clinical Medicine*, 2(3), 374-380. https://doi.org/10.4236/ijcm.2011.23066

5. Samuelsen, A. B. (2000). The traditional uses, chemical constituents and biological activities of *Plantago major L.* A review. *Journal of Ethnopharmacology*, 71(1-2), 1-21. https://doi.org/10.1016/S0378-8741(00)00212-9

6. Zhang, Y., Xu, S., Liang, R., & Mao, X. (2011). Aucubin inhibits the apoptosis induced by hydrogen peroxide in PC12 cells. *European Journal of Pharmacology*, 657(1-3), 121-127. https://doi.org/10.1016/j.ejphar.2011.01.062

7. Natural Medicines Comprehensive Database. (2021). Plantain. Retrieved from https://naturalmedicines.therapeuticresearch.com

Poria

1. Bensky, D., & Gamble, A. (1993). *Chinese Herbal Medicine: Materia Medica* (Revised ed.). Eastland Press.

2. Chen, H., Zhang, Q., Wang, X., & Yang, L. (2018). Anti-inflammatory and immunomodulatory effects of Poria cocos. *International Journal of Molecular Sciences*, 19(10), 1705. https://doi.org/10.3390/ijms19101705

3. Li, X., He, X., Li, S., Chen, W., Sun, J., & Zhang, J. (2014). Chemical composition and antioxidant activities of the essential oil from Poria cocos. *Chemistry Central Journal*, 8(1), 9. https://doi.org/10.1186/1752-153X-8-9

4. Li, X., Wang, Q., Yang, G., & Zhao, X. (2015). Traditional Chinese medicine in treatment of diabetic peripheral neuropathy: A systematic review and meta-analysis. *Journal of Traditional Chinese Medicine*, 35(6), 696-704. https://doi.org/10.1016/S0254-6272(16)30067-2

5. Liu, B., Zhang, X., Wang, X., & Shen, G. (2016). Effect of Poria cocos polysaccharides on peripheral nerve regeneration in rats with sciatic nerve injury. *Journal of Ethnopharmacology*, 194, 98-106. https://doi.org/10.1016/j.jep.2016.09.037

6. Wang, K., Bao, L., Xiong, W., Ma, K., Han, L., & Zhang, H. (2017). Immunomodulatory function of a polysaccharide purified from Poria cocos mycelia in immunosuppressed mice. *International Journal of Biological Macromolecules*, 96, 681-686. https://doi.org/10.1016/j.ijbiomac.2016.12.054

7. Zhang, J., Gao, Y., & Zhou, S. (2019). Neuroprotective effects of Poria cocos polysaccharides on oxidative stress-induced apoptosis in PC12 cells. *International Journal of Biological Macromolecules*, 129, 844-852. https://doi.org/10.1016/j.ijbiomac.2019.02.072

Quercetin

1. Zeng, X., Cai, W., & Li, J. (2019). Quercetin ameliorates high glucose-induced Schwann cell damage by reducing oxidative stress and improving mitochondrial function. Neural Regeneration Research, **14**(11), 2102–2108. DOI:10.4103/1673-5374.262584
2. Chen, W., Yang, C., & Huang, H. (2015). Bioavailability and Pharmacokinetics of Quercetin: A Review. Journal of Food and Drug Analysis, **23**(2), 157–169. DOI:10.1016/j.jfda.2014.10.001
3. Oyagbemi, A. A., Saba, A. B., & Azeez, O. I. (2010). Molecular targets of quercetin in cancer management. African Journal of Traditional, Complementary and Alternative Medicines, **7**(3), 187–195. DOI:10.4314/ajtcam.v7i3.54777
4. Pal, R., Vaiphei, K., & Mahmood, A. (2014). Neuroprotective effects of quercetin in diabetic neuropathy: A morphometric study. Intractable & Rare Diseases Research, **3**(1), 23–31. DOI:10.5582/irdr.2014.01005
5. D'Andrea, G. (2015). Quercetin: A flavonol with multifaceted therapeutic applications? Fitoterapia, **106**, 256–271. DOI:10.1016/j.fitote.2015.09.018
6. Li, Y., Yao, J., Han, C., Yang, J., Chaudhry, M. T., Wang, S., Liu, H., & Yin, Y. (2016). Quercetin, Inflammation and Immunity. Nutrients, **8**(3), 167. DOI:10.3390/nu8030167
7. Anand David, A. V., Arulmoli, R., & Parasuraman, S. (2016). Overviews of Biological Importance of Quercetin: A Bioactive Flavonoid. Pharmacognosy Reviews, **10**(20), 84–89. DOI:10.4103/0973-7847.194044

Sumac

1. Esmaeili, M. A., & Yazdanparast, R. (2004). Hypoglycaemic effect of *Rhus coriaria* L. (sumac) fruits extract in streptozotocin-induced diabetic rats. *Phytotherapy Research*, 18(6), 454–457. https://doi.org/10.1002/ptr.1472

2. Gul, U. D., Acıkara, Ö. B., Sevimli-Gür, C., Erdoğan Orhan, İ., & Savaşer, A. (2017). *Rhus coriaria* L.: Evaluation of its chemical composition and antioxidant activity. *Journal of Pharmacy and Pharmacology*, 69(9), 1198–1206. https://doi.org/10.1111/jphp.12754

3. İlahı, G., Küpeli Akkol, E., Süntar, İ., & Keleş, H. (2020). Evaluation of anti-inflammatory and antinociceptive activities of sumac (*Rhus coriaria* L.). *Journal of Ethnopharmacology*, 253, 112646. https://doi.org/10.1016/j.jep.2020.112646

4. Jalali, M. T., Mahmoodi, M., Zarshenas, M. M., & Mokhtari, S. (2020). Efficacy of sumac (*Rhus coriaria* L.) powder on glycemic control and insulin resistance in type 2 diabetic patients: A randomized, double-blind, placebo-controlled clinical trial. *Journal of the American College of Nutrition*, 39(5), 424–429. https://doi.org/10.1080/07315724.2020.1729403

5. Kosar, M., Bozan, B., Temelli, F., & Baser, K. H. C. (2007). Antioxidant activity and phenolic composition of sumac (*Rhus coriaria* L.) extracts. *Food Chemistry*, 103(3), 952–959. https://doi.org/10.1016/j.foodchem.2006.09.051

6. Mohammadhosseini, M., Sarker, S. D., & Akbarzadeh, A. (2017). Chemical composition of the essential oils and extracts of *Rhus coriaria* L. and their biological activities: A review. *Iranian Journal of Basic Medical Sciences*, 20(4), 451–468. https://doi.org/10.22038/IJBMS.2017.8678

7. Pourahmad, J., Eskandari, M. R., Shakibaei, R., Kamalinejad, M., & Minaiyan, M. (2010). Protective effects of *Rhus coriaria* against sodium arsenite-induced acute hepatotoxicity in rats. *Archives of Industrial Hygiene and Toxicology*, 61(4), 303–309. https://doi.org/10.2478/10004-1254-61-2010-2013

8. Zare, K., Ebrahimi, L., Karimi, E., & Oskoueian, E. (2019). A review on antioxidant, anti-inflammatory, and antimicrobial properties of *Rhus coriaria* and its bioactive compounds. *International Journal of Food Properties*, 22(1), 1626–1641. https://doi.org/10.1080/10942912.2019.1650753

TB-500

1. https://www.peptidesciences.com/blog/thymosin-beta-4-neuropathy-senescence
2. https://www.peptides.org/tb-500-side-effects/
3. https://calbizjournal.com/tb500-and-pain-management-alleviating-discomfort-through-regeneration/
4. https://www.peptidesciences.com/blog/tb-500-and-the-brain

THC

1. Hampson, A. J., Grimaldi, M., Axelrod, J., & Wink, D. (1998). Cannabidiol and (−)Δ9-tetrahydrocannabinol are neuroprotective antioxidants. *Proceedings of the National Academy of Sciences*, 95(14), 8268-8273. https://doi.org/10.1073/pnas.95.14.8268
2. Mackie, K. (2008). Cannabinoid receptors: where they are and what they do. *Journal of Neuroendocrinology*, 20(s1), 10-14. https://doi.org/10.1111/j.1365-2826.2008.01671.x
3. Nagarkatti, P., Pandey, R., Rieder, S. A., Hegde, V. L., & Nagarkatti, M. (2009). Cannabinoids as novel anti-inflammatory drugs. *Future Medicinal Chemistry*, 1(7), 1333-1349. https://doi.org/10.4155/fmc.09.93
4. Pertwee, R. G. (2008). The diverse CB1 and CB2 receptor pharmacology of three plant cannabinoids: Δ9-tetrahydrocannabinol, cannabidiol and Δ9-tetrahydrocannabivarin. *British Journal of Pharmacology*, 153(2), 199-215. https://doi.org/10.1038/sj.bjp.0707442
5. Russo, E. B. (2007). History of cannabis and its preparations in saga, science, and sobriquet. *Chemistry & Biodiversity*, 4(8), 1614-1648. https://doi.org/10.1002/cbdv.200790144
6. Russo, E. B. (2008). Cannabinoids in the management of difficult to treat pain. *Therapeutics and Clinical Risk Management*, 4(1), 245-259. https://doi.org/10.2147/tcrm.s1928
7. Wallace, M. S., Marcotte, T. D., Umlauf, A., Gouaux, B., & Atkinson, J. H. (2015). Efficacy of inhaled cannabis on painful diabetic neuropathy. *The Journal of Pain*, 16(7), 616-627. https://doi.org/10.1016/j.jpain.2015.03.008

Vitamin B12

1. https://onlinelibrary.wiley.com/doi/pdfdirect/10.1111/cns.13207
2. https://www.mdpi.com/1422-0067/25/1/590
3. https://www.mdpi.com/2072-6643/12/8/2221
4. https://www.invigormedical.com/immune-health/vitamin-b12-for-nerve-pain/

5. https://practicalneurology.com/articles/2020-mar-apr/peripheral-neuropathy-caused-by-vitamin-b12-deficiency

Vitamin B6

1. https://www.mdpi.com/2072-6643/15/13/2823
2. https://jps.biomedcentral.com/articles/10.1007/s12576-019-00659-8
3. https://www.hsa.gov.sg/announcements/safety-alert/high-dose-vitamin-b6-and-risk-of-peripheral-neuropathy
4. https://link.springer.com/article/10.1007/s40264-018-0664-0
5. https://www.foundationforpn.org/wp-content/uploads/2022/01/Stewart_Vitamin-B6_J-Peripheral-Nervous-Sys_2021.pdf

White Mulberry

1. Asano, N., Yamashita, T., Yasuda, K., Ikeda, K., Kizu, H., Kameda, Y., Kato, A., Nash, R. J., Lee, H. S., & Ryu, K. S. (2001). Polyhydroxylated alkaloids isolated from mulberry trees (Morus alba L.) and silkworms (Bombyx mori L.). Journal of Agricultural and Food Chemistry, 49(9), 4208–4213. **Journal of Agricultural and Food Chemistry**
2. Kim, S. Y., Gao, J. J., Lee, W. C., Ryu, K. S., Lee, K. R., & Kim, Y. C. (2000). Antioxidative flavonoids from the leaves of Morus alba. Archives of Pharmacal Research, 23(4), 426–430. **Archives of Pharmacal Research**
3. El-Beshbishy, H. A., & Singab, A. N. (2006). Hypolipidemic and antioxidant activities of Morus alba L. (Egyptian mulberry) root bark extracts in streptozotocin-induced diabetic rats. Life Sciences, 78(23), 2724–2733. **Life Sciences**
4. Asai, A., Nakagawa, K., Higuchi, O., Kimura, T., Kojima, Y., Nagao, A., & Kiso, Y. (2011). Novel alpha-glucosidase inhibitors from natural products: suppression of postprandial hyperglycemia by mulberry leaves. Journal of Nutritional Science and Vitaminology, 57(3), 224–227. **Journal of Nutritional Science and Vitaminology**
5. Wattanathorn, J., Muchimapura, S., Thukham-Mee, W., Wannanon, P., Tong-Un, T., & Wannanon, P. (2012). Mulberry fruits mitigate neuropathic pain in chronic constriction injury model rats. American Journal of Applied Sciences, 9(7), 1012–1018. **American Journal of Applied Sciences**
6. Lown, M., Fuller, R., Lightowler, H., Fraser, A., Gallagher, A., Stuart, B., Byrne, C. D., & Lewith, G. (2017). Mulberry extract lowers the glycaemic index of white bread in healthy human volunteers: A pilot study. Nutrition Research, 44, 1–8. **Nutrition Research**
7. National Center for Complementary and Integrative Health. (2016). Mulberry Leaf. **NCCIH - Mulberry Leaf**

www.ingramcontent.com/pod-product-compliance
Lightning Source LLC
Chambersburg PA
CBHW061031250726
48653CB00001B/53